Management
OF
Countertransference
WITH
Borderline Patients

Management

OF

Countertransference

WITH

Borderline Patients

Glen O. Gabbard, M.D.

Professor of Psychiatry
Baylor College of Medicine
Training and Supervising Analyst
The Houston-Galveston Psychoanalytic Institute
Houston, Texas

Sallye M. Wilkinson, Ph.D.

Private Practice in
Clinical Psychology and Psychoanalysis
Topeka, Kansas

Washington, DC 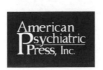 London, England

American
Psychiatric
Press, Inc.

Note: The authors have worked to ensure that all information in this book concerning drug dosages, schedules, and routes of administration is accurate as of the time of publication and consistent with standards set by the U.S. Food and Drug Administration and the general medical community. As medical research and practice advance, however, therapeutic standards may change. For this reason and because human and mechanical errors sometimes occur, we recommend that readers follow the advice of a physician who is directly involved in their care or the care of a member of their family.

Books published by the American Psychiatric Press, Inc., represent the views and opinions of the individual authors and do not necessarily represent the policies and opinions of the Press or the American Psychiatric Association.

Copyright © 1994 American Psychiatric Press, Inc.
ALL RIGHTS RESERVED
Manufactured in the United States of America on acid-free paper
04 03 02 01   6 5 4 3
First Edition

American Psychiatric Press, Inc.
1400 K Street, N.W., Washington, DC   20005

Library of Congress Cataloging-in-Publication Data
Gabbard, Glen O.
    Management of countertransference with borderline patients / Glen
O. Gabbard, Sallye M. Wilkinson. — 1st ed.
        p.   cm.
    Includes bibliographical references and index.
    ISBN 0-88048-563-9
    1. Borderline Personality Disorder—Treatment.
2. Countertransference (Psychology).   I. Wilkinson, Sallye M.
II. Title.
    [DNLM: 1. Countertransference (Psychology).   2. Borderline
Personality Disoder—therapy.   3. Psychotherapy—methods.   WM 62
G112m 1994]
RC569.5.B67G33   1994
616.85′8520651—dc20
DNLM/DLC
for Library of Congress   93-47462
                                                                                   CIP

British Library Cataloguing in Publication Data
A CIP record is available from the British Library.

Digitally printed at Edwards Brothers Digital Book Center

To the memory of
Jean Collmus Wilkinson
and
T. D. Wilkinson III

Contents

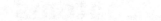

Source Acknowledgments

The authors gratefully acknowledge permission to reprint portions of the following material:

Gabbard GO: "Splitting in Hospital Treatment." *American Journal of Psychiatry* 146:444–451, 1989. Copyright 1989, the American Psychiatric Association. Portions reprinted with permission in Chapter 8.

Gabbard GO: "Technical Approaches to Transference Hate in the Analysis of Borderline Patients." *International Journal of Psychoanalysis* 72(4):625–637, 1991. Copyright Institute of Psycho-Analysis, London, 1991. Portions reprinted with permission in Chapter 5.

Gabbard GO: "The Therapeutic Relationship in Psychiatric Hospital Treatment." *Bulletin of the Menninger Clinic* 56(1):4–19, 1992. Copyright 1992, the Menninger Foundation. Portions reprinted with permission in Chapter 8.

Gabbard GO: "An Overview of Countertransference With Borderline Patients." *Journal of Psychotherapy Practice and Research* 2(1):7–18, 1993. Copyright 1993, American Psychiatric Press, Inc. Portions reprinted with permission in Chapter 1.

Wilkinson SM, Gabbard GO: "Therapeutic Self-Disclosure With Borderline Patients." *The Journal of Psychotherapy Practice and Research* 2:282–295, 1993. Copyright 1993, American Psychiatric Press, Inc. An expanded version of this article appears with permission as Chapter 7.

Introduction

Few disorders in psychiatry would warrant an entire volume devoted to the emotional reactions they generate in the clinicians who treat them. Borderline personality disorder is unique in its capacity to stir up affects that overwhelm treaters. In the best of circumstances, the feelings activated in the treatment of such patients provide crucial data about the patient's internal world that may help to resolve a treatment impasse. In the worst of circumstances, the countertransference evoked in the treatment may compel clinicians to pursue ill-advised courses of action that result in unethical boundary transgressions by the therapist or suicide attempts by the patient.

In the course of conducting seminars throughout the country on the treatment of borderline patients, we have been struck by the ravages of countertransference in mental health professionals who treat borderline patients. The personal and professional lives of those clinicians are affected in an extraordinary way. Some clinicians describe being "driven crazy" by such patients. Others feel their personal lives have been so invaded that they must tell their children not to answer the telephone when it rings. Still others have vowed never to treat another borderline patient because they "simply can't take it anymore."

The book we have written is designed to address the emotional tempest that therapists who treat borderline patients must face. We have provided a systematic approach to examining and managing the myriad countertransference reactions that arise in the course of treatment. We have chosen to illustrate this approach by reporting detailed accounts of the minute-by-minute and hour-by-hour interaction between therapist and patient. Although the management of countertransference is only one aspect of the overall treatment of persons with borderline personality disorder, it is clear that no other part of the treatment can be carried out in the manner intended if the clinician's emotional reactions are not taken into account first.

Treatment of borderline patients has a long and distinguished tradition at The Menninger Clinic. Indeed, the very notion of the borderline patient originated in the seminal writings of Robert Knight when he worked at The Menninger Clinic in the 1950s. During the 1960s and early 1970s, while Otto Kernberg was director of the C. F. Menninger Memorial Hospital, his classic papers on the concept of borderline personality organization were published. In the last two decades, borderline patients have been referred to The Menninger Clinic from all over the world, and groups of clinicians and researchers have continued to devote much of their careers to the understanding and treatment of these difficult-to-treat patients.

Our collaboration as coauthors of this volume began as a supervisor-supervisee relationship. As the two of us mutually struggled to articulate a methodology with which to approach the overwhelming emotional reactions encountered in the psychotherapy of borderline patients, the mentor-mentee nature of the relationship evolved over a period of a few years into a collegial collaboration. We first presented material at the 1991 annual meeting of the American Psychiatric Association in New Orleans in the Continuous Clinical Case Seminar format. The overflow crowd and the enthusiasm of the audience in attendance convinced us that our work should be expanded to monograph form. We have designed the book to be useful to both experienced and beginning therapists of all professional disciplines.

Writing about countertransference requires an uncompromising honesty. Although we have disguised clinical material so that patients are not recognizable, we have tried to be as open as possible about our own feelings that we encountered in the course of our work. We are grateful to a number of our Menninger colleagues who graciously shared some of their feelings in specific cases that we discussed with them. Many of their struggles also appear on the pages of this volume. The difficult self-revelation required by these accounts will be well worth it if other clinicians find them enriching and useful in their own work.

Faye Schoenfeld's superb typing and editing shaped the final form of the manuscript, and Claire Reinburg's assistance at American Psychiatric Press in the development of this project was much appreciated. Finally, we would like to express appreciation to our spouses, Joyce Davidson Gabbard and George Hough, for their patience and support through the extended process of taking this project from an idea to its ultimate end point.

CHAPTER 1

Overview of Countertransference With Borderline Patients

I feel used/manipulated/abused and at the same time feel responsible for her feelings of rejection and threats of suicide, or feel made to feel responsible for them because I don't have time for her, and I don't choose/cannot be always available as a good object, nor as a stand-by part object.

She has hooked me into thinking love/friendship will heal her, as if there is nothing wrong with her, but that it is all of the people in her life who are the problem. Then I come up with fatherly friendship, and her control begins. She tells me, in different ways, that I am different than the others. And just when I'm basking in "good objectivity," she really begins to control me by telling me that I'm just like the rest, I don't care: "I see you looking at your watch. I know you want to leave. I know you have a life out there. It will be a long night. You don't care. Nobody cares."

As this quotation from a borderline patient's therapist vividly conveys, patients with borderline personality disorder tend to overwhelm the clinicians that treat them. A comprehensive treatment program for such patients often includes individual psychotherapy or psychoanalysis, adjunctive pharmacotherapy with any one of a number of agents, brief or extended hospitalization, family or marital therapy, and group psychotherapy. Regardless of the specific form of treatment, however, countertransference can be a major impediment to successful therapeutic efforts (Boyer 1990). The treater's emotional reactions to the patient sweep through the course of treatment like a veritable tempest with the potential to decimate both patient and therapist in its wake. Although the skillful management of countertransference is only one aspect of an overall treatment approach to borderline personality disorder, it constitutes the foundation of the treatment on which all other efforts will rise or fall.

The primitive defenses of borderline patients, particularly splitting and projective identification, produce a kaleidoscopic array of complex and chaotic transferences in the therapeutic setting. As these varying configurations of self- and object-representations parade before the therapist, they are further complicated by accompanying affect states that are unusually intense and raw, often inducing in therapists a feeling that they are trapped in a life-and-death struggle (Kernberg et al. 1989). Some clinicians have even suggested that countertransference reactions may be the most reliable guide to making the diagnosis of borderline personality disorder (Solomon et al. 1987). They make us "come alive" in a specific way that heightens our awareness much like the experience of driving over a mountain pass on a narrow, two-lane road without a guard rail. Because they are so sensitive to the therapist's choice of words and nonverbal nuances, they are able to evoke a sense of "walking on eggshells," as though our margin of error is very narrow indeed. Yet, despite this untoward impact, they somehow become "special" to their therapists (Gabbard 1986) and inspire a surprising optimism despite a host of pessimistic prognostic signs (Solomon et al. 1987). Therapeutic zeal rises like a phoenix from the ashes of previous failures.

Borderline patients seem to have the peculiar ability to inflict a specific form of "sweet suffering" on their therapists. They themselves have suffered throughout their lives, and it is important to them to have their therapists suffer for them (Giovacchini 1975). They seem to demand that the therapist abandon the professional therapeutic role so that whoever attempts to treat them must share in their misery. Searles (1986) cautioned that the traditional analytic posture of evenly suspended attention is neither viable nor appropriate in the psychotherapy of borderline patients. Therapists who attempt to assume a detached, "objective" role vis-à-vis the borderline patient are at risk for projectively disavowing their own conflicts and anxieties and using the patient as a container to receive them. The classical notion of the therapist as "blank screen" is simply not applicable in the same way to the psychotherapy of borderline patients.

Specific Countertransference Reactions

Controversy over the diagnosis of borderline personality disorder persists despite the introduction of this category into DSM-III (American Psychiatric Association 1980) 14 years ago. The first systematic empirical study of the disorder by Grinker and colleagues (1968) suggested that borderline personality disorder is a spectrum that ranges from the psychotic to the neurotic. Kernberg (1967, 1975) argued that the borderline concept is really a personality organization rather than a specific nosological entity. A variety of different personality disorders, including paranoid, antisocial, schizoid, infantile, narcissistic, and cyclothymic, all could be subsumed under the overarching ego organization.

Gunderson (1984), on the other hand, sought to identify discriminating criteria that would distinguish borderline personality disorder from other related Axis II conditions. Abend and colleagues (1983) raised serious questions about the Kernberg (1967) diagnostic understanding of borderline patients by documenting the successful psychoanalytic treatment of such patients with classical psychoanalytic technique based on traditional conflict theory. Adler (1985) presented yet another point of view. He proposed that borderline patients could best be understood as suffering from a deficit-based condition rather than intrapsychic conflict. Specifically, this condition involved the absence of a holding-soothing introject that could sustain them emotionally in the absence of their psychotherapists. Other clinicians influenced by self psychology (Brandchaft and Stolorow 1987; Terman 1987) maintained that borderline symptomatology results from breakdowns in the empathic relatedness between therapist and patient and should therefore be reconceptualized as an entity that is definable only in the context of a relationship.

This controversy about diagnosis is mirrored in a corresponding controversy regarding the optimal treatment. Much (although not all) of the differences of opinion can be accommodated by embracing Meissner's (1988) notion that the borderline diagnosis is essentially a spectrum of conditions that are psychodynamically related. At the "high" end of the spectrum are patients who have notable ego strengths and can undergo psychoanalytic treatment with little modification. At the "low" end of the spectrum are patients prone to psychotic disorganization because of prominent ego weaknesses and who require more supportive approaches.

However, from a clinical perspective, the spectrum must be regarded as a metaphorical construct. Borderline patients are known for wide fluctuations in their clinical presentation. One can see normal, neurotic, and psychotic transferences in the same patient in the course of one therapeutic hour (Little 1958). A corollary of this observation is that therapists must assume a *flexible* approach to the psychotherapy, where their interventions shift to and fro along the expressive-supportive continuum according to the patient's needs at a particular moment. Meissner (1988) shared this point of view and offered the following observation:

> My own view is that, while the theoretical discrimination between supportive and expressive modalities has a certain utility from the point of view of articulating and describing aspects of the psychotherapeutic process, attempts to hold rigidly to a dichotomous view that prescribes a given form of therapeutic modality to specific diagnostic entities is neither theoretically sustainable nor clinically practical . . . the therapist needs to maintain a position of flexibility and adaptability, allowing the selection of available techniques from the range of psychotherapeutic interventions to deal with the problems presented. (p. 121)

The conceptual framework of a spectrum is important because in discussions of countertransference, one must keep in mind that the therapist's reactions may vary considerably, depending on where a particular patient resides on the continuum from the lowest-level group to the higher-level patients. Meissner (1988) observed that "countertransference in relation to borderline conditions is therefore not an univocal phenomenon but rather involves a spectrum of levels and intensities of transference/countertransference interactions that can vary considerably in both quality and quantity" (p. 211). With this caveat in mind, we consider several common countertransference reactions to borderline patients.

Guilt Feelings

Borderline patients possess an uncanny ability to tune in to the therapist's vulnerabilities and exploit them in a manner that induces feelings of guilt. A common development is that a patient will behave in such a way as to infuriate and exasperate the therapist. At the very moment the therapist is wishing the patient would disappear, the patient may accuse the therapist of not caring and disliking the patient. Such accusations may create feelings in therapists that they have been "found out." Under such conditions therapists may reproach themselves for their lack of professionalism and attempt to make amends to their patients by professing undying devotion. The patient's accusatory charges may strike to the very marrow of the therapist's professional identity and create a form of "physiological countertransference" (Gabbard 1986) that involves manifestations of sympathetic discharge, such as a pounding heart, a dry mouth, and trembling limbs.

Another common scenario is that the therapist begins to feel responsible for apparent clinical deterioration in the course of psychotherapy. Many borderline patients appear relatively intact at the beginning of treatment and seem to unravel as therapy progresses. Searles (1986) suggested that such guilt may be related to unconscious empathy with the patient's child self-representation, who felt guilty about driving a parental figure to the point of madness. He noted also that some therapists will feel guilty that the patient's more psychotic aspects provide greater fascination than the healthier or more neurotic areas of the ego.

Rescue Fantasies

Intimately related to guilt feelings are the evocation of rescue fantasies in the therapist. This aspect of the countertransference involves more than simply therapeutic zeal. It also reflects a perception that the patient is essentially helpless. Therapists often feel that they must do things *for* the patient. Borderline patients often present themselves like orphaned waifs out of a Dickens novel (Gabbard 1986), who therefore need the therapist to serve as a "good" mother or father to make up for the "bad" or absent parent responsible for victimizing the child.

Transgressions of Professional Boundaries

The third form of specific countertransference reaction follows naturally from the first two. Borderline patients are notorious for evoking deviations from the therapeutic frame that lead to ill-advised boundary crossing (Eyman and Gabbard 1991; Gutheil 1989, 1991). These patients may present with a specific form of entitlement resulting in demands to be treated as exceptions to the usual procedures. They are known to have a "short fuse" that leads to frequent expressions of rage. The origins of this proneness to primitive expressions of aggression may be constitutional (Kernberg 1975) or secondary to trauma (Herman et al. 1989), but the end result is that therapists often feel threatened or intimidated by the patient's volatility and potential to explode.

To ward off the patient's anger, the therapist may extend the session, engage in self-disclosure, defer payment or not charge any fee whatsoever, or engage in physical or sexual behavior with the patient. In some cases, this violation of professional boundaries is rationalized because of the perception of the patient as a victim who is entitled to compensation in the form of extraordinary measures because of the suffering endured. Suicide threats may also lead therapists to justify various forms of boundary transgressions, often with the claim that if they had not deviated from their usual practices, the patient would have committed suicide (Eyman and Gabbard 1991).

Still another source of boundary transgressions relates to the issue of abandonment. Many borderline patients feel that they are always on the verge of being abandoned by significant sources of nurturance and support, typically their parents, lovers, or therapists (Masterson and Rinsley 1975; Rinsley 1989). Some patients interpret any communication from the therapist—except unconditional love—as having an implicit threat of rejection (Adler 1985). These patients' demands for reassurance that one really cares and is not simply a prostitute who receives a fee in return for time and attention may lead therapists to go to extraordinary lengths to demonstrate their sincere concern. Because these demands may escalate to late-night phone calls, a rendezvous outside the therapy, and sexual liaisons, therapists who treat borderline patients have an ethical as well as a clinical need to understand countertransference pitfalls thoroughly (Chessick 1977).

Rage and Hatred

A common element in the psychotherapy of borderline patients is ridding themselves of tension by evacuating or "dumping" feelings into the therapist (Boyer 1990), what Rosenfeld (1987) termed a "lavoratoric transference." Whereas neurotic patients tend to project superego constellations into the therapist, borderline patients project the "sick" or "bad" self in a primitive split-off form (Boyer 1987; Kernberg 1975; Volkan 1987). In other words, *part* self- and object-representations are "dumped" into the therapist, resulting in a pressure to identify unconsciously with aspects of the patient that represent two-dimensional extremes. The therapist may feel "all bad" or thoroughly hateful without any sense of good or loving feelings to temper the extreme negative passions. This experience of becoming a part object frequently leads the therapist to feel that an alien force is taking over from within (i.e., one is not acting like oneself). Volkan described the feeling of being "choked" by the externalization of such primitive and negatively charged affects and introjects. One can hardly avoid feeling rage, hatred, and resentment when being used as a "toilet" by the patient. Being held hostage to suicide threats or being driven to distraction by late-night phone calls and unceasing demands for extraordinary treatment can also lead to profound feelings of seething resentment.

Helplessness and Worthlessness

Borderline patients tend to devalue their therapists' efforts (Adler 1985). Also, when their demands are frustrated rather than gratified, these patients can shift from idealizing to contemptuous transferences in the twinkling of an eye. They tend to indulge in *pars pro toto* thinking in which one becomes "all bad" for even a minor transgression. The result is that therapists often feel "deskilled," incompetent, and helpless to do anything about it. This form of countertransference is further enhanced by the expertise of borderline patients at identifying vulnerable areas and exploiting that awareness by constantly pointing out weaknesses to the therapist. Defensiveness and withdrawal are often overt postures of the therapist in the throes of such devaluing attacks, but underneath the surface the feelings of helplessness and incompetence are prominent.

Anxiety and Terror

Regardless of what else is going on in the treatment, borderline patients almost always make the therapist anxious. The sources of this anxiety are many and varied. At the most primitive level, the borderline patient's confusion about boundaries may lead therapists to feel a primal terror related to the concern that they will be swallowed up by their patient and annihilated. In psychotic transferences, patients may misidentify feelings belonging to them as residing in the therapist instead. A feeling of merger or fusion may be extremely unsettling to the therapist in such situations. The anxiety that the patient will commit suicide is ever present in many treatment processes, and the sense of guilt and responsibility induced by the patient makes such worries amplified as compared with other patients. The previously mentioned concern that one will say the wrong thing and cause the patient to explode, fragment, or walk out of the office abruptly also creates countertransference anxiety. Finally, an overriding anxiety that runs throughout the treatment is the feeling that therapists often have that they are simply not up to the clinical task or are failing in their efforts.

The Nature of Countertransferences

As the concept of countertransference has moved squarely to center stage in contemporary psychoanalytic discourse, it has undergone a transformation in its meaning. Countertransference as a disruptive obstacle has been replaced by a view of countertransference as a valuable, if not essential, source of understanding. Accompanying this shift is heightened interest in how the patient-therapist relationship serves as a forum for reenactments of past experiences. The archaeological search for the buried past has been replaced by careful attention to the moment-by-moment reverberations between therapist and patient (Lester 1990).

Freud's (1910/1957) original definition of countertransference was narrowly focused on the analyst's transference to the patient. In other words, countertransference involved feelings that belonged to the analyst's past but were displaced onto the patient in the same way that the patient displaced feelings from the past onto the analyst. This view conceptualized countertransference as an interference or obstacle that needed to be removed by rigorous analysis of the analyst.

Heimann (1950) altered the landscape of psychoanalytic thinking. In her view, countertransference needed to be construed in a much broader form as *all* the feelings that the analyst experiences toward the patient.

Implicit in Heimann's (1950) broad or totalistic understanding of countertransference was the notion that some of the feelings the analyst experiences are *induced* by the patient's behavior. Racker (1968) divided such reactions into concordant and complementary countertransferences. Concordant countertransferences are those involving an empathic link between therapist and patient (i.e., the therapist identifies with the patient's subjective affective state or self-representations). Complementary countertransferences involve identifications with an internal object-representation of the patient that has been projectively disavowed and attributed to the therapist. Racker viewed this complementary reaction as an instance in which the analyst's own conflicts were activated by the patient's projections. Grinberg (1979) took this notion one step further with the concept of projective counteridentification, in which the analyst introjects a reaction, feeling, or object-representation that comes *entirely* from the patient.

Winnicott (1949), in his classic paper on countertransference hate, spoke of an "objective" form of countertransference in which the analyst reacted to the patient in a specific manner evoked by the patient that was consistent across all people who interacted with the patient. According to this schema, certain patients might consistently induce feelings of hate in other people that reflect more about the patient than about the analyst's or other person's past.

This shift in thinking led to an outpouring of interest in the Kleinian concept of projective identification (Boyer 1987, 1990; Gabbard 1994; Goldstein 1991; Grotstein 1981; Kernberg 1975, 1987; Ogden 1979, 1982; Porder 1987; Sandler 1987b; Scharff 1992; Searles 1986; Tansey and Burke 1989). Although the original concept as used by Klein (1946/1975) involved an intrapsychic fantasy rather than an interpersonal coercion, the modern usage has focused to a great extent on changes in the recipient of the patient's projective identification. Whereas the concept remains highly controversial, there is a general consensus that the split-off self-representation, object-representation, or affect that the patient projects into the therapist produces changes in the therapist to conform to the nature of that projection.

These changes are effected largely through powerfully coercive interpersonal pressure exerted by the patient. Projective identification, as one of the central defense mechanisms employed by borderline patients, takes on crucial importance for our discussion, and we elaborate on it later in this chapter.

One implication of this shift in thinking about countertransference is that the analyst's response to the patient provides a great deal of information about the patient's internal object world. Moreover, countertransference entails serving as a container to receive projected aspects of the patient and studying the contents of those projections. Sandler (1976) suggested that the analyst's free-floating attention must be supplemented by a free-floating responsiveness involving a form of introspection that determines what complementary role is being coerced by the patient's words and behavior.

This influence from the British school of object relations theory has traveled across the Atlantic and has had a significant impact on the classical or ego-psychological school in the form of considerable interest in concepts such as interaction and enactment (Chused 1991; Coen 1992; Jacobs 1986, 1991; McLaughlin 1991). In an overview of countertransference and technique, Abend (1989) acknowledged that the notion originating with Klein that the analyst's countertransference can be a crucial source of understanding the patient's inner world has now become universally accepted. As part of this acceptance, the self-analytic activities of the analyst have come to be regarded as a systematic effort at collecting data about one's analysand. The analyst must be particularly attuned to subtle or not-so-subtle forms of "acting in," whereby the patient's internal object relationships are enacted in the clinical setting between patient and analyst. In speaking of enactments, Chused (1991) noted:

> An analyst reacts to his patient—but catches himself in the act, so to speak, regains his analytic stance, and in observing himself and the patient, increases his understanding of the unconscious fantasies and conflicts in the patient and himself which have prompted him to action. (p. 616)

Borderline patients, in particular, evoke enactments through the sheer power of the affect and the primitive self- and object-representations that are projected into the therapist. However, it would be erroneous to assume that all of an analyst's countertransference reactions are simply aspects of the patient. In our view, countertransference must be thought of as a *joint creation,* in which both the therapist's past conflicts and the patient's projected aspects create specific patterns of interaction within the therapeutic process. Indeed, a central feature of the therapist's role with such patients is to engage in an introspective process that attempts to differentiate one's own contributions from those of the patient (Gabbard 1994; Kernberg et al. 1989). Bollas (1987) noted that "in order to find the patient we must look for him within ourselves. This process inevitably points to the fact that there are 'two patients' within the session and therefore two complementary sources of free association" (p. 202). The therapist, then, must maintain both an intrapsychic focus and an interpersonal focus in an effort to sort out what is going on within the patient and bear it within himself or herself (Coen 1992).

If one accepts the premise that countertransference is a joint creation, it also follows that the relative contributions of therapist and patient vary according to the severity of the psychopathology. In general, projective identification or "objective" countertransferences occur with sicker patients, such as those suffering from borderline personality disorder, whereas the narrow or "subjective" countertransferences are more prominent with healthier or neurotic patients. Although many countertransference reactions with borderline patients are overwhelming in intensity, we must not neglect more elusive forms of enactment that also occur throughout the spectrum of psychopathology. Jacobs (1991) pointed out that even aspects of the standard analytic or therapeutic posture, such as neutrality or silence, can become involved in subtle enactments that are unconsciously determined by issues in both patient and therapist.

This modernization of the concept of countertransference has led some to believe that the term has been expanded so greatly that it has lost a certain specificity in meaning. Natterson (1991), for example, made a differentiation between countertransference and the therapist's own subjectivity. He preferred the language of "intersubjectivity" because the therapist initiates as well as reacts. However, in actual practice the interactions between therapist and patient are so inextricably bound up with one another that what is initiative and what is reactive may be next to impossible to dissect.

Meissner (1988) also argued for a narrower or more limited view of countertransference. In his view, not all reactions that the therapist experiences toward the patient should be construed as countertransference. He proposed that only the analyst's transference to the patient and the analyst's reaction to the role assigned by the patient should be regarded as countertransference. In this conceptualization, certain reactions involve the real relationship of patient and therapist and the therapeutic alliance. Again, this distinction may be extremely difficult to tease out in the heat of the affective storms generated by borderline patients in psychotherapy.

The conceptualization of countertransference that we are advocating in this book places great responsibility on therapists to see themselves as both clinicians and as "patients" whose own issues enter into the therapeutic arena (Bollas 1987, 1990; Boyer 1987; Searles 1986). Self-analysis, then, is of paramount importance in effectively managing countertransference. Indeed, Bollas (1990) observed that "my view . . . is that contemplation of the countertransference is a systematic reintegration into the psychoanalytical movement of an exiled function: that of self-analysis" (p. 339).

The Role of Projective Identification

In light of the central importance of projective identification in the psychotherapy of borderline patients and in the conceptualization of countertransference as we have defined it, a more careful consideration may be helpful in clarifying our use of this term in subsequent chapters. Despite the controversy over the confusing usages of the term, we view the concept as essential for understanding the transference-countertransference developments in psychotherapy of patients with borderline personality disorder.

To begin with, projective identification should be regarded as more than simply a defense mechanism of borderline patients. Ogden (1979) defined it as a three-step procedure in which the following events occur. First, an aspect of the self is projectively disavowed by unconsciously placing it in someone else. Second, the projector exerts interpersonal pressure that coerces the other person to experience or identify unconsciously with what has been projected. Third, the recipient of the projection (in the therapeutic situation) processes and contains the projected contents leading to a reintrojection of them by the patient in modified form. Ogden also stressed that the projector feels a sense of oneness or union with the recipient of the projection.

This model transcends the simple purpose of defense. As Scharff (1992) eloquently summarized, four distinct purposes can be identified for projective identification:

> (1) Defense: to distance oneself from the unwanted part or to keep it alive in someone else, (2) Communication: to make oneself understood by pressing the recipient to experience a set of feelings like one's own, (3) Object-relatedness: to interact with a recipient separate enough to receive the projection yet undifferentiated enough to allow some misperception to occur to foster the sense of oneness, and (4) Pathway for psychological change: to be transformed by reintrojecting the projection after its modification by the recipient, as occurs in the mother-infant relationship, in marriage, or the patient-therapist relationship. (p. 29)

This model of projective identification carries with it a spirit of therapeutic optimism. If therapists can bear the projections of their patients, they offer the hope of helping patients transform their internal world through containment and modification of those projections and affects in the crucible of the therapist's countertransference. Some critics of this model (Kernberg 1987; Sandler 1987a) objected, arguing that Ogden (1979) broadened the definition beyond Klein's (1946/1975) original intent by including the third step involving reintrojection. Kernberg preferred to regard projective identification as a primitive defense mechanism involving projecting intolerable aspects of the self, maintaining empathy with the projected contents, attempting to control the object, and unconsciously inducing the object to play the role of what is projected in the actual interaction between the projector and the recipient.

Sandler (1987a) also objected to extending the projective identification concept to include the therapeutic actions of containment, detoxification, and modification as described by Ogden (1979). However, Sandler's (1976) notion of role responsiveness is very much in keeping with the first two steps of Ogden's concept and with our view of countertransference as joint creation of patient and therapist. He stated:

> Very often the irrational response of the analyst, which his professional conscience leads him to see entirely as a blind spot of his own, may sometimes be usefully regarded as a compromise-formation between his own tendencies and his *reflexive acceptance of the role which the patient is forcing on him.* (p. 46)

Of those who write about projective identification, most agree that control is a central feature of the process. Patients may experience that the depositing of aspects of themselves in the therapist forges a powerful link between the two members of the dyad, giving them the illusion of influence over the therapist. Often the power of this control is recognized only after the therapist has responded in the specific manner that has been unconsciously programmed by the patient's projective identification. Therapists of borderline patients must accept that countertransference enactments or "acting out" is inevitable. By rigorously monitoring internal responses, therapists can at least regroup and process what has happened with the patient following such enactments.

Boyer (1982) also construed projective identification broadly in the manner of Ogden (1979). In fact, he wrote that the patient's reintrojection of what has been projected into the therapist is a neglected aspect of the process. When they project hostility, for example, into their therapists, these patients may benefit by the "detoxification" of the affect and associated self- or object-representation through the therapist's containment process. Boyer believed that an important therapeutic element of projective identification is the patient's observation that neither therapist nor patient is destroyed by the projection and reintrojection of negative affects.

Although Scharff (1992) shared the broadened view of projective identification that we are endorsing, she stressed that the patient and therapist engage in a mutual process. Moreover, she placed greater emphasis on the introjective identification component of the therapist who receives aspects of the patient. The therapist may respond in a concordant or complementary manner, according to Racker's (1968) distinction, but Scharff also noted that introjective identification is determined in part by the therapist's own propensity to respond in an identificatory manner with what is projected by the patient. In other words, some projections may represent a "good fit," whereas others may be experienced as alien and discarded. Finally, Scharff observed that the reintrojective process by the patient-projector may promote change if the containment by the therapist-recipient has made slight modifications that can be accepted within the limits of the patient's capacity to change.

This can also be pathological, however, if the projection is returned in a completely distorted form that does not modify the patient's anxiety or lead to psychological change. Certainly in nontherapeutic settings the aspects that are projected are routinely "crammed back down the patient's throat" rather than contained or modified, often with considerably intensified affect. The expanded model of projective identification assumes a therapeutic context in which containment and modification are goals. (It should be noted that close friends, parents, lovers, spouses, and the like may also be "therapeutic" in the way they contain what has been projected into them even though a formal psychotherapy process is not involved.)

The joint creation model of countertransference that we believe is most apposite for the psychotherapy of borderline patients depends heavily on the expanded model of projective identification as described by Ogden (1979), Boyer (1990), Scharff (1992), and others. It is of crucial importance, however, that therapists keep in mind the *metaphorical* nature of the exchange of mental contents. There is nothing mystical about projective identification. When patients coerce us into specific behaviors or feelings that correspond with what they have projected into us, they have simply stimulated repressed or split-off aspects of ourselves just as troops far from the front may be called into service when specific forms of battle need to be fought. We all possess a myriad of self-representations that are integrated into a more or less continuously experienced sense of self. We all have sadists and murderers lurking in our depths as well as saints and heroes. Considerable insight is gained in conceptualizing the psychotherapeutic process as involving "two patients," rather than one, by understanding that the most bizarre aspect of the patient has some parallel counterpart in ourselves (Searles 1986).

In reflecting on the challenge of treating borderline patients, Lewin and Schulz (1992) made the following observation:

> What makes us so uncomfortable in the face of the patient's pressures on us is not what is in the patient but what is in ourselves that corresponds to what comes from the patient. . . . In treating borderline patients and others with severe character disorders, the most dangerous character disorder is our own. In fact, a definition of working with borderline patients that stated the central task for the therapist was getting to know aspects of himself that he did not wish to know would make good sense, provided that it emphasized that the therapist might be discomfited to find himself not only worse than he had thought himself to be but also better. (p. 119)

The Role of Theory

Francis Bacon once said that even wrong theories are better than chaos. Our attention to theory in this chapter emphasizes that theoretical models are perhaps most useful when struggling with intense countertransference feelings. They bring order to the chaos of overwhelming affect and intense transference distortions. Friedman (1988) noted that the practice of psychotherapy involves considerable discomfort for the psychotherapist a good deal of the time. One dimension of the application of theory to the clinical situation is that it also is applying balm to soothe the therapist's anxiety.

Nevertheless, one must never regard theory as absolute or allow it to become reified. Theories are only as valuable as their clinical utility. Although we have borrowed from object relations theory in our conceptualization of countertransference, and specifically projective identification, other theoretical models have been used to explain the same clinical phenomena. Porder (1987) shared Ogden's (1979) view that projective identification is not simply a defense mechanism. However, he explained it from a traditional ego-psychological perspective. Projective identification, in Porder's view, is an identification with the aggressor that is a chronic repetition of an entrenched pattern of relatedness between child and parent. The patient achieves active mastery over a passively experienced trauma by unconsciously casting the analyst in the role of the child while the patient assumes the parental role. In Porder's model, the affect is not projected into the analyst; it is simply induced by the patient.

Adler and Rhine (1988) approached projective identification from a self psychological perspective. Kohut (1971, 1977, 1984) stressed the need for the therapist to serve as a selfobject to the patient. In other words, therapists must allow themselves to be used by the patient for psychological growth. The therapist's selfobject functions include allowing mirroring, idealization, and twinship in the patient's transferences. Adler and Rhine described a case of a patient who insisted that her therapist function as a selfobject by accepting her provocations and projections. They pointed out that the containing and modifying aspect of projective identification converges with selfobject functioning in situations where the therapist understands and tolerates the need to be used by the patient and helps the patient verbalize feelings rather than acting on them. Different theories, the authors suggested, are essentially struggling with the same clinical issues.

Most therapists use multiple models (Gabbard 1994; Pine 1990; Sandler 1990). Rigid adherence to only one theoretical frame when the clinical data do not fit the theory is an unfortunate phenomenon in contemporary practice that privileges theory over clinical observation. Theory can also be misused to rationalize counter-transference acting out (Chessick 1977). One can use self psychology to rationalize enjoyment of idealization by a patient. Similarly, one can misuse Kernberg's (1975) encouragement to confront and interpret the negative transference early on in the therapy to justify expressions of anger at the patient. Bollas (1989) stressed that modern analysts must understand a variety of analytic schools: "The psychoanalyst is an object performing multiple functions, each analyst-object being significantly more present than another ana-

lyst-object according to the clinical requirements of the analysand"
(p. 100).

Summary

Just as the borderline diagnosis falls along a spectrum, the
therapist's countertransference also reflects a continuum of responses. The primitive defenses of borderline patients, particularly
splitting and projective identification, contribute to a pattern of intense, chaotic, and potentially problematic countertransference reactions. Prominent among these countertransference responses
are guilt feelings, rescue fantasies, transgressions of professional
boundaries, rage and hatred, helplessness, worthlessness, anxiety,
and even terror. With patients who are as primitively organized as
those suffering from borderline personality disorder, the broad or
totalistic view of countertransference is perhaps more useful than
the narrow Freudian notion. Projective identification is one way of
systematically understanding how aspects of the patient's internal
world come to be experienced by the therapist. However, all of a
therapist's feelings in relation to a patient cannot necessarily be
attributed to the patient's projective processes. Whether or not a
projection "takes" is also related to whether it is a good fit with the
therapist's preexisting internal object world. Therefore, countertransference must always be viewed as a *joint creation,* in which both
the therapist's past conflicts and the patient's projected aspects create specific patterns of interaction within the therapeutic process.
Although projective identification has emerged from Kleinian theory, analysts writing from ego-psychological and self psychological
perspectives have described much the same phenomena with
slightly different formulations.

References

Abend SM: Countertransference and psychoanalytic technique. Psycho-
    anal Q 48:374–395, 1989

Abend SM, Porder MS, Willick MS: Borderline Patients: Psychoanalytic Perspectives. New York, International Universities Press, 1983

Adler G: Borderline Psychopathology and Its Treatment. New York, Jason Aronson, 1985

Adler G, Rhine MW: The selfobject function of projective identification: curative factors in psychotherapy. Bull Menninger Clin 52:473–491, 1988

American Psychiatric Association: Diagnostic and Statistical Manual of Mental Disorders, 3rd Edition. Washington, DC, American Psychiatric Association, 1980

Bollas C: The Shadow of the Object: Psychoanalysis of the Unthought Known. New York, Columbia University Press, 1987

Bollas C: Forces of Destiny: Psychoanalysis and Human Idiom. Northvale, NJ, Jason Aronson, 1989

Bollas C: Regression in the countertransference, in Master Clinicians on Treating the Regressed Patient. Edited by Boyer LB, Giovacchini PL. Northvale, NJ, Jason Aronson, 1990, pp 339–352

Boyer LB: Analytic experiences in work with regressed patients, in Technical Factors in the Treatment of the Severely Disturbed Patient. Edited by Giovacchini PL, Boyer LB. New York, Jason Aronson, 1982, pp 65–106

Boyer LB: Regression and countertransference in the treatment of a borderline patient, in The Borderline Patient: Emerging Concepts in Diagnosis, Psychodynamics, and Treatment, Vol 2. Edited by Grotstein JS, Solomon MF, Lang JA. Hillsdale, NJ, Analytic Press, 1987, pp 41–47

Boyer LB: Countertransference and technique, in Master Clinicians on Treating the Regressed Patient. Edited by Boyer LB, Giovacchini PL. Northvale, NJ, Jason Aronson, 1990, pp 303–324

Brandchaft B, Stolorow RD: The borderline concept: an intersubjective viewpoint, in The Borderline Patient: Emerging Concepts in Diagnosis, Psychodynamics, and Treatment, Vol 2. Edited by Grotstein JS, Solomon MF, Lang JA. Hillsdale, NJ, Analytic Press, 1987, pp 103–125

Chessick RD: Intensive Psychotherapy of the Borderline Patient. New York, Jason Aronson, 1977

Chused JF: The evocative power of enactments. J Am Psychoanal Assoc 39:615–639, 1991

Coen SJ: The Misuse of Persons: Analyzing Pathological Dependency. Hillsdale, NJ, Analytic Press, 1992

Eyman JR, Gabbard GO: Will therapist-patient sex prevent suicide. Psychiatric Annals 21:651–655, 1991

Freud S: The future prospects of psycho-analytic therapy (1910), in The Standard Edition of the Complete Psychological Works of Sigmund Freud, Vol 11. Translated and edited by Strachey J. London, Hogarth Press, 1957, pp 139–151

Friedman L: The Anatomy of Psychotherapy. Hillsdale, NJ, Analytic Press, 1988

Gabbard GO: The treatment of the "special" patient in a psychoanalytic hospital. International Review of Psychoanalysis 13:333–347, 1986

Gabbard GO: Psychodynamic Psychiatry in Clinical Practice: The DSM-IV Edition. Washington, DC, American Psychiatric Press, 1994

Giovacchini PL: Tactics and Techniques in Psychoanalytic Therapy, Vol 2: Countertransference. New York, Jason Aronson, 1975

Goldstein WN: Clarification of projective identification. Am J Psychiatry 148:153–161, 1991

Grinberg L: Countertransference and projective counteridentification, in Countertransference. Edited by Epstein L, Feiner AH. New York, Jason Aronson, 1979, pp 169–191

Grinker Jr RR, Werble B, Drye RC: The Borderline Syndrome: A Behavioral Study of Ego-Functions. New York, Basic Books, 1968

Grotstein JS: Splitting and Projective Identification. New York, Jason Aronson, 1981

Gunderson JG: Borderline Personality Disorder. Washington, DC, American Psychiatric Press, 1984

Gutheil TG: Borderline personality disorder, boundary violations, and patient-therapist sex: medicolegal pitfalls. Am J Psychiatry 146:597–602, 1989

Gutheil TG: Patients involved in sexual misconduct with therapists: is a victim profile possible? Psychiatric Annals 21:661–667, 1991

Heimann P: On counter-transference. Int J Psychoanal 31:81–84, 1950

Herman JL, Perry JC, van der Kolk BA: Childhood trauma in borderline personality disorder. Am J Psychiatry 146:490–495, 1989

Jacobs TJ: On countertransference enactments. J Am Psychoanal Assoc 34:289–307, 1986

Jacobs TJ: The Use of the Self: Countertransference in the Analytic Situation. Madison, CT, International Universities Press, 1991

Kernberg OF: Borderline personality organization. J Am Psychoanal Assoc 15:641–685, 1967

Kernberg OF: Borderline Conditions and Pathological Narcissism. New York, Jason Aronson, 1975

Kernberg OF: Projection and projective identification: developmental and clinical aspects, in Projection, Identification, Projective Identification. Edited by Sandler J. Madison, CT, International Universities Press, 1987, pp 93–115

Kernberg OF, Selzer MA, Koenigsberg HW, et al: Psychodynamic Psychotherapy of Borderline Patients. New York, Basic Books, 1989

Klein M: Notes on some schizoid mechanisms (1946), in Envy and Gratitude and Other Works, 1946–1963. New York, Delacorte, 1975, pp 1–24

Kohut H: The Analysis of the Self: A Systematic Approach to the Psychoanalytic Treatment of Narcissistic Personality Disorders. New York, International Universities Press, 1971

Kohut H: The Restoration of the Self. New York, International Universities Press, 1977

Kohut H: How Does Analysis Cure? Edited by Goldberg A. Chicago, IL, Chicago University Press, 1984

Lester EP: Gender and identity issues in the analytic process. Int J Psychoanal 71:435–444, 1990

Lewin RA, Schulz CG: Losing and Fusing: Borderline and Transitional Object and Self Relations. Northvale, NJ, Jason Aronson, 1992

Little M: On delusional transference (transference psychosis). Int J Psychoanal 39:134–138, 1958

Masterson JF, Rinsley DB: The borderline syndrome: the role of the mother in the genesis and psychic structure of the borderline personality. Int J Psychoanal 56:163–177, 1975

McLaughlin JT: Clinical and theoretical aspects of enactment. J Am Psychoanal Assoc 39:595–614, 1991

Meissner WW: Treatment of Patients in the Borderline Spectrum. Northvale, NJ, Jason Aronson, 1988

Natterson J: Beyond Countertransference: The Therapist's Subjectivity in the Therapeutic Process. Northvale, NJ, Jason Aronson, 1991

Ogden TH: On projective identification. Int J Psychoanal 60:357–373, 1979

Ogden TH: Projective Identification and Psychotherapeutic Technique. New York, Jason Aronson, 1982

Pine F: Drive, Ego, Object, and Self: A Synthesis of Clinical Work. New York, Basic Books, 1990

Porder MS: Projective identification: an alternative hypothesis. Psychoanal Q 56:431–451, 1987

Racker H: Transference and Countertransference. New York, International Universities Press, 1968

Rinsley DB: Developmental Pathogenesis and Psychoanalytic Treatment of Borderline and Narcissistic Personalities. Northvale, NJ, Jason Aronson, 1989

Rosenfeld H: Impasse and Interpretation: Therapeutic and Anti-Therapeutic Factors in the Psychoanalytic Treatment of Psychotic, Borderline, and Neurotic Patients. London, Tavistock, 1987

Sandler J: Countertransference and role-responsiveness. International Review of Psychoanalysis 3:43–47, 1976

Sandler J: The concept of projective identification, in Projection, Identification, Projective Identification. Edited by Sandler J. Madison, CT, International Universities Press, 1987a, pp 13–26

Sandler J (ed): Projection, Identification, Projective Identification. Madison, CT, International Universities Press, 1987b

Sandler J: On internal object relations. J Am Psychoanal Assoc 38:859–880, 1990

Scharff JS: Projective and Introjective Identification and the Use of the Therapist's Self. Northvale, NJ, Jason Aronson, 1992

Searles HF: My Work With Borderline Patients. Northvale, NJ, Jason Aronson, 1986

Solomon MF, Lang JA, Grotstein JS: Clinical impressions of the borderline patient, in The Borderline Patient: Emerging Concepts in Diagnosis, Psychodynamics, and Treatment, Vol 1. Edited by Grotstein JS, Solomon MF, Lang JA. Hillsdale, NJ, Analytic Press, 1987, pp 3–12

Tansey MJ, Burke WF: Understanding Countertransference: From Projective Identification to Empathy. Hillsdale, NJ, Analytic Press, 1989

Terman DM: The borderline concept: a critical appraisal and some alternative suggestions, in The Borderline Patient: Emerging Concepts in Diagnosis, Psychodynamics, and Treatment, Vol 1. Edited by Grotstein JS, Solomon MF, Lang JA. Hillsdale, NJ, Analytic Press, 1987, pp 61–71

Volkan VD: Six Steps in the Treatment of Borderline Personality Organization. Northvale, NJ, Jason Aronson, 1987

Winnicott DW: Hate in the counter-transference. Int J Psychoanal 30:69–74, 1949

CHAPTER 2

Establishment of Optimal Distance

Throughout the course of psychotherapy with borderline patients, therapists may feel that they are engaged in an ongoing struggle to maintain their professional role and identity. Many patients with borderline personality disorder convey either explicitly or subtly that something other than a psychotherapeutic relationship is what they really need. Therapists may feel they are under powerful pressure to cross boundaries by extending sessions, not charging a fee, disclosing aspects of their personal lives, or engaging in physical contact. Alternatively, because of these pressures, they may become overly rigid and distant toward the patient to ensure that no ethical transgressions will occur. Establishing and maintaining optimal distance in the therapeutic relationship, therefore, is one of the primary challenges facing the therapist.

Especially during the opening phase of the treatment, therapists may feel that the boundaries of the relationship are tested repeatedly. A sense of floundering is a common experience while searching for an appropriately therapeutic atmosphere. Therapists may feel overwhelmed with the patient's wish to establish a relationship that in no way resembles psychotherapy. Often the boundary testing comes in a remarkably concrete form, as illustrated by the following:

> In the first session of psychotherapy, Ms. Z entered Dr. A's office, and Dr. A offered her a chair at the side of his desk. Ms. Z proceeded to sit down and scoot the chair across the floor until it was

next to Dr. A's desk chair. Ms. Z had relocated the chair in such a way that when she sat, her knee was actually touching Dr. A's knee. The therapist immediately felt intruded upon, anxious, and a bit off balance by this unexpected development. Ms. Z immediately began to launch into an account of her problems without any apparent recognition of Dr. A's discomfort.

Dr. A did nothing for a few moments as he contemplated his options. Should he simply tolerate this encroachment to indicate his flexibility and empathy with the patient's needs? Should he slide his chair back away from the patient? Would such a decision result in devastating consequences for Ms. Z's self-esteem? Should he ask her to return her chair to its original location?

After considering the various options, Dr. A recognized that he was too uncomfortable to achieve the optimal state of mind necessary for conducting psychotherapy. He said to Ms. Z: "I don't want to hurt your feelings, but I would feel much more comfortable if you returned your chair to its usual place." The patient acceded to his request without protest and continued talking. Later exploration in psychotherapy revealed that Ms. Z had been an incest victim and had never really established generational boundaries in her own family. An attempt to reestablish a boundariless situation in psychotherapy was thus natural for her.

In this vignette the establishment of optimal distance involved a literal, spatial distance. Dr. A used his countertransference anxiety to recognize that his inability to enter into a psychotherapeutic space was directly related to the lack of physical space between the patient and him. Processing his feelings and requesting to restore physical distance in the relationship helped Dr. A regain psychological distance and a sense of control and mastery over the situation. More often, however, the issue of distance is a symbolic, psychological one rather than a concrete, physical one, as in the following case example:

Ms. Y entered Dr. B's office for her first session and stared for a moment or two at her therapist. She looked disappointed and even irritated.

Dr. B: I take it that I don't look like what you expected.

Ms. Y: No! I wanted someone older. Someone to mother me. Someone like Ellen, my last therapist. [Ms. Y begins to cry.] You look younger than I am. I know you are!

Dr. B was uncomfortably aware that she was actually a few years younger than the patient. Despite her attempt to be objective about this nagging awareness, the therapist had a vague feeling that she should apologize to the patient. As she speculated about why she might be feeling that way, she invited further elaboration from Ms. Y about her wish for "mothering" and her feelings about her last therapist.

Ms. Y: Ellen gave me this necklace I'm wearing. [She stroked the beads.] It used to be hers.
Dr. B: So you feel like she's with you.
Ms. Y: She was like a mother to me for 2 years. Now I'm not with her because my husband had to change jobs and move here. [Ms. Y cries profusely.]

Dr. B felt as if Ms. Y had been wrenched unjustly from the only person in the world who could possibly help her. She began to doubt if she would ever measure up to this idealized figure.

Ms. Y: I sold my collection of rare stamps so I could be in therapy with Ellen. Those stamps were the most valuable things we owned. But I sold them because Ellen was my life. I had no money left, so I arranged to work at a convenience store so I could be in the neighborhood where Ellen lives. But the people I worked for didn't appreciate my sensitivity to allergens. When I started to be unable to go to work, they put a lot of pressure on me. I was in and out of hospitals for a while, and most of the doctors wouldn't okay passes for me to go to Ellen's office for therapy. They thought I would kill myself. But not as long as I was with Ellen! I would *never* do that as long as I was with her. One doctor during one of my hospitalizations let me go to Ellen's office. Once I was there, I couldn't leave. I wouldn't leave. It became a bit of a problem.

Dr. B knew that the patient had refused to leave her previous therapist's office on many occasions. For some reason this detail made an extraordinarily strong impression on Dr. B. In fact, she had noted that, even prior to this first session, she had already been aware of anxiety connected with the fantasy that she would have to pry the patient from her office at the end of the hour. As Ms. Y spoke, the therapist took note of how the patient minimized her own contributions to her presenting problems.

Ms. Y: Did you know that I have severe TMJ? It's horrible. I suffer constantly. My head feels strange, and I can't function. I didn't know that I had it until Ellen diagnosed it. Since she helped me discover it, I've been to many holistic health doctors. I've tried herbs and altered my diet. Now I'm taking medication. It's the only way that I can survive.

The patient became increasingly tearful and was soon gasping for air because she was crying so hard. Dr. B, without the benefit of a shared history with the patient, wondered what would come next. With growing anxiety, she waited to see what the patient would do.

Ms. Y [still gasping for air between sobs]: Ellen knows me so well! We are like mother and child. She rearranged the furniture in her office so I would be comfortable. She knows me so well. She used to say she's keeping all of the parts of me, and then one day we'll put it all back together. Now I'm here, and she has all of me back there!

Dr. B felt it was necessary to begin to establish herself as the patient's therapist. She began to grow weary of all the focus on Ellen and wanted to reorient the patient's attention to the difficulties she was having entering a relationship with her.

Dr. B: You are here, and yet you're not here.

Ms. Y: Ellen is so wonderful. There's no way for me to tell you all that she knows. I could never tell you what I've told her. She knows about my mother, my husband, and my fear of people. Ellen said she'd be there for me always. If I could be with her, everything would be okay.

Dr. B: Have you written to her?

Ms. Y: No! I'm angry with her for referring me to you! She said she couldn't help me any more. She said she'd always be there, and she left me! If she left me, that means other people can do it too!

Dr. B [empathizing with how the patient's anger had turned to anguish]: So what you are feeling is that much worse!

Ms. Y: Yes. That kind of match will never happen again.

Dr. B: I don't know about that. I think with new people there are always uncertainty and worries and fears. But uncertainty is not the same as "no possible match."

Ms. Y: I saw Ellen three or four times a week for 2 years. We did *good* work together. I ended up in the hospital and couldn't see her. All I wanted was to get back to her. I talked to Ellen on the phone every day. Ellen told me that she couldn't help me on the phone. So I did *everything* I could do to get well enough to go back to Ellen. I sold everything. I ran out of money. But I finally got back to Ellen. Finally, all I had to do was take the bus to Ellen's office, but I couldn't leave her. I wouldn't leave at the end of the session. Then something happened to change me about 4 months ago. I haven't been able to do anything since. I'm afraid to go out. I can't work. I've been disconnected with people—even Ellen—since then. Ellen noticed a change in me, and she called it *borderline* [spitting out "borderline" as if it were an unthinkable insult].

Dr. B: Disconnected? Meaning withdrawn? Or feeling disconnected inside?

Ms. Y: Inside.

Dr. B observed that the patient described this inner "disconnectedness" as if it were equivalent to the social isolation about which she also complained. Dr. B's anxiety skyrocketed as she soberly noted to herself that Ms. Y seemed to assume that it was the therapist's job to resolve both types of difficulties for her. Clearly, the patient expected Dr. B to resolve *all* of her difficulties. The therapist felt that she was being inordinately pressured to make a deal. She also had a sinking feeling that she could not possibly be adequate to the task. Moreover, the therapist knew that if she promised anything to the patient, the result would be disastrous because the patient would inevitably be disappointed. Dr. B began to realize that the intense pressured experience could be understood as something that was being "dumped" from the patient into her through the process of projective identification. She was then able to intervene from an empathic perspective.

Dr. B: You must feel a great deal of pressure right now.

Ms. Y [nodding affirmatively, pausing thoughtfully for a few moments]: Things didn't work out too well with Ellen. I might as well die if I'm going to suffer like this. I can't live without Ellen. I have to get better to get back to her. I keep looking for Ellen here. I know I get delusional at times. Ellen told me that I do. I know she's not here. But I look for her, and I hope I'll see someone like her here who will be my therapist.

Dr. B: You're right of course. Ellen is not here. But she seems to be with you in the necklace you're wearing.

Ms. Y: Yes. But I'm not real good at keeping people with me inside. Something in there eats them up.

Dr. B: It's fortunate that you understand how that works in you. Some people only suffer and never know why. You seem to have some understanding of your suffering.

Ms. Y: Yes, I do. I don't even know your name. I can't remember. I know your first name. Can I call you that?

For a moment, Dr. B wanted to say yes. She wanted to be as good as Ellen had been and inspire the confidence in Ms. Y that her previous therapist had. However, she caught herself in the midst of this wish to gratify and decided to stick to her typical professional boundaries.

Dr. B: I prefer to be called "Dr. B."

Ms. Y: When I was with Ellen, there were times when I just wanted to suck on her breast. We would talk about that. Ellen explained to me that that is how things go wrong between a little baby and her mother. I thought it was weird when she first said those things—about sucking on breasts and all. But she explained to me how it worked. Ellen said that I had trouble with dependency.

Dr. B: There are about 10 minutes left. I wasn't sure if you wanted to comment on our talk so far or talk about what comes next.

Dr. B recognized that she was anxious to address the end of the hour because she felt overwhelmed by the dependency longings in the patient concretized in the form of a wish to suck her previous therapist's breast. She was continuing to harbor the fantasy that the patient might refuse to leave her office. She was concerned that the patient's sobbing would complicate the end of the hour, and she wanted to bring the session to a gradual completion.

Ms. Y: You seem awfully young. Younger than me. I equate youth with inexperience. Ellen was more experienced than you. She taught at the medical school.

Dr. B: What you know of me is what you see, and you're uncertain what I have inside of me.

Ms. Y: Yes—you are young. I knew it.

Dr. B [slightly ruffled and a bit annoyed]: You have yet to become familiar with who I am on the inside.

Ms. Y: We haven't decided how often we'll meet. I brought this letter from Ellen for you. May I read it? This is her handwriting. Isn't it lovely?

The therapist listened as the patient read the entire seven-page letter. Ellen expressed feelings of affection and compassion toward Ms. Y. She offered reassuring statements that the patient would always be important to her. Ellen suggested to Ms. Y that she needed four psychotherapy sessions a week plus the opportunity to make up to 10 phone calls a week if she were in crisis.

Dr. B heard the letter as a cautionary tale about the difficulties of future work with Ms. Y. The prospect of being available to the patient through numerous sessions and phone calls each week felt overwhelming. In addition to her reluctance to attempt to offer the patient more than she knew that she could deliver, Dr. B felt hesitant to compete with such a highly idealized object. Based on a diagnostic understanding of the patient's need to develop further the ego strength necessary to sustain her between sessions, as well as the patient's need to mourn the loss of this idealized figure who functioned as an external prop to her internal world, Dr. B decided to offer the patient two sessions per week.

Ms. Y: That's what she wrote. I know the time is up now.

Dr. B: Yes, it is. Thank you for sharing the letter. I suggest that we meet twice a week.

Ms. Y: That would be fine. Is there any possibility we could meet three times a week?

Dr. B: Let's get started first. Later, we can talk about that possibility. It's time to stop for today. [The patient leaves very slowly.]

This excerpt from the beginning of a psychotherapy process can be used to illustrate a number of the issues involved in establishing optimal distance during the opening phase of therapy.

Confusion and Uncertainty

Within moments of meeting Ms. Y, Dr. B was plunged into a state of chaos, ambiguity, and confusion. Her anxiety escalated as Ms. Y informed her that she was too young. The patient began to sob as an expression of her disappointment. The previous therapist, Ellen, was held up as an impossible standard—one that Dr. B could never hope to match. Additionally, Ms. Y presented the relationship as a mother-child situation rather than a psychotherapeutic encounter. Dr. B felt overwhelmed by the sense of desperation Ms. Y conveyed when she described her previous therapeutic relationship. The immersion in this intense affective experience is an essential and unavoidable aspect of the psychotherapy with borderline patients. Bollas (1987) described it well: "The [analyst's] most ordinary countertransference state is a not-knowing-yet-experiencing one" (p. 203).

The therapist needs to tolerate this experience without feeling the need to organize all the material immediately into a coherent conceptual framework. Moreover, prematurely interpreting the primitive transference that is being observed can be a technical error. At the outset of therapy the transference is a more general one to the unknown qualities of the therapist (Casement 1990). Often such early interventions may grow out of a countertransference need to gain immediate ideational mastery over the intense affect and may be viewed by the patient as too general or even hostile.

As one tolerates the transference-countertransference chaos of the process, a pattern usually emerges that sheds considerable light on the difficulty establishing optimal distance. Borderline patients tend to oscillate between twin dangers (Lewin and Schulz 1992). On the one hand, attachment brings with it the fear of merger, with the accompanying loss of self. On the other hand, borderline patients fear that if they allow too much distance, they will then lose the therapist. These dual dangers place borderline patients on the horns of a dilemma—if they defend against the anxiety about fusing with the object, they are then thrust into the opposite danger of being isolated from the object they so desperately need. The result is an oscillating pattern of clinging followed by retreat. The therapist's countertransference responses mirror these shifts between oscillating poles. As Lewin and Schulz (1992) noted, "either there is overidentification with the patient or there is complete unempathic rejection. The first aggravates the fusion danger for the patient. The second accentuates the loss danger" (p. 79). Both members of the therapeutic dyad struggle to find some sense of middle ground in the context of what seems like an obligatory all-or-none situation.

One way to view the therapist's intense affective state and the sense of floundering accompanying that state is that the patient has created an "illness" in the therapist. Dr. B's mounting anxiety about whether Ms. Y would leave the office, whether she would fall apart, and whether she would be able to engage in a psychotherapeutic process made her feel pressured to act in some manner to relieve the anxiety. Much of her efforts were directed more at management of her own anxiety than at the patient's presenting concerns. Bollas (1987) acknowledged this aspect of therapy by commenting that therapists must often treat their own situational illnesses before being able to treat those of the patient. By extension, the therapist is also treating the patient's illness as it manifests itself in the induction of certain states in the therapist.

Time Urgency

Throughout the course of psychotherapy, but particularly in the early phases, many borderline patients will present their problems as though they require emergency attention involving some form of drastic action by the therapist. This presentation creates a sense of countertransference urgency that makes the therapist feel as though the patient cannot possibly wait until understanding of the situation can be achieved through psychological exploration. The heaving sobs of Ms. Y made Dr. B feel as though a catastrophe was occurring that would not be amenable to ordinary psychotherapeutic interventions.

Many borderline patients spend a great deal of time functioning in a paranoid-schizoid mode of thinking. In this psychological constellation, there is no subjective "I," no sense of self that involves personal agency that extends over time (Ogden 1986). Patients operating in this mode live in "the now," with no recall of times in the past when they were able to survive experiences of intense affective pain or emptiness. The notion of delaying gratification of their needs is also dismissed as unthinkable because the future seems irrelevant and unconnected to the immediate sense of urgency. One central feature of splitting as a defense mechanism is that self-experiences are kept in a kind of psychic limbo where they remain unconnected with other self-experiences. There is no continuous thread woven between the needy, desperate self and the quiet, contented self so that the two experiences of being can be integrated into a complex, continuous self-experience.

The kind of overwhelming despair that patients like Ms. Y bring to a psychotherapy hour is powerfully compelling. A psychological emergency is apparently taking place and requires immediate attention. This affectively powerful self-presentation may coerce a complementary object response in the therapist through the process of projective identification. The object response that "possesses" the therapist is that an action outside the conventional therapeutic role is needed to address the emergency. The patient may need to be physically held. The next hour may need to be canceled so the therapist can remain with the patient. The patient may seem to require medication to regain control. A third party (a boss or spouse, for example) may need to be called so the therapist can intervene on the patient's behalf.

A consideration of the sense of time urgency engendered by borderline patients leads naturally into a discussion of pharmacotherapy. One survey of psychiatrists in private practice who were experienced in the psychodynamic psychotherapy of borderline patients (Waldinger and Frank 1989) revealed that 90% of them prescribed medication at some point in the treatment of borderline patients. A recurrent issue for such psychotherapists, however, is to monitor whether the decision to prescribe grows out of countertransference exasperation or solid clinical judgment.

A rational and systematic approach to prescribing for borderline patients is essential to avoid ill-advised pharmacotherapy out of a sense of despair or a need to "do something." For thorough discussions of the pharmacotherapy of borderline personality disorder, see Soloff (1993) and Cowdry and Gardner (1988).

Feelings of Inadequacy

From the first moments of Ms. Y's encounter with Dr. B, she induced feelings of inadequacy in her therapist. She was dismayed at the relative youth of Dr. B. She was reduced to tears when she compared Dr. B with her previous therapist. Dr. B's reaction to her own awareness of the age comparison was to feel guilty and to contemplate making an apology to the patient. This reaction, which the therapist noted as irrational, is a typical development in the psychotherapy of borderline patients. They are masters at inducing feelings of guilt about things for which the therapist should feel no compunction whatsoever.

Having had a string of therapists is common for patients with borderline personality disorder because they move from one clinician to another, always hoping that their needs will finally be gratified in a magical manner by a particularly special therapist. Hence, previous therapists are frequently invoked in either idealized or devalued terms by these patients. In the case of Ms. Y, her previous therapist, Ellen, was regarded as nothing short of a savior. As the number of superlatives applied to the previous therapist mounted, Dr. B felt increasingly futile about ever being able to live up to this paragon of therapeutic virtuosity. A key element in this aspect of the countertransference was Ms. Y's portrayal of her clinical improvement as totally outside her own control. Only what the therapist does matters. Dr. B felt that she could not possibly measure up to Ellen, so her ability to help the patient was severely limited. These feelings of being inadequate and "deskilled" dislodged the therapist from her professional role and made her feel helpless to influence the course of the session.

For therapists to react defensively in such situations in an effort to assert their own competence vis-à-vis the previous therapist is understandable. Another common countertransference response is to compete with the previous therapist by becoming more active, more interpretive, or more gratifying than therapists ordinarily would be in a first session. Some may also respond with contempt or disdain for the actions of the previous therapist. Borderline patients often tell stories about the extraordinarily special relationship they had with their therapists. Although some of these accounts may well be accurate, caution should be used in accepting such reports at face value. In many instances, including Ms. Y's account of Ellen, the previous therapist will insist that the accounts are heavily contaminated by transference wishes.

The Wish for Parenting

Another characteristic of the paranoid-schizoid mode of functioning is a collapse of "analytic space," which Ogden (1986) defined as "the space between patient and analyst in which analytic experience (including transference illusion) is generated and in which personal meanings can be created and played with" (p. 238). One result of this phenomenon is that borderline patients will often view the psychotherapist literally as though he or she were a parent. The "as if" nature of the psychotherapeutic relationship is lost and requires an opening of analytic space so that the therapist can be viewed as like a parent but still different. Ogden (1986) noted, "the therapist working with borderline patients is forever attempting to 'pry open' the space between symbol and symbolized, thus creating a field in which meanings exist, where one thing stands for another in a way that can be thought about and understood" (p. 241). The wish for parenting can then be reflected on and examined as an idea worth understanding.

In the absence of this capacity, the patient may relate to the therapist in the same manner described in the first session with Ms. Y. She did not enter into the therapeutic relationship with the expectation of working through problems with her actual mother by reexperiencing those issues with a new object. Instead, she literally expected the therapist to be a mother to her. She was devastated that Dr. B was so young because she was afraid she would not be mothered by her therapist. She then went on to give an account of her previous therapist that made it appear as though Ellen actually served as a mother in her life. The most dramatic example of this concretization of the transference wish was her comment that she wanted to suck Ellen's breast.

This striking loss of psychological distance creates profound countertransference reactions that are likely to disarm a therapist during the opening phase. Dr. B felt overwhelmed by the intense dependent longings expressed by Ms. Y. She felt as though she were being swallowed up by her patient's voracious need for succor. She also felt deskilled, as though her technical expertise and training were of no use to the patient. The patient's crushing disappointment made Dr. B feel as though she would need to be an idealized "good mother" to be of any help whatsoever to the patient.

Although Ms. Y's demands for parenting were "up front" in the beginning of the process, other borderline patients may not explicitly ask for a parental relationship but unconsciously expect unconditional loving responses from the therapist and react with rage when they do not receive it. An advantage of Ms. Y's presentation was that the transference wish was out on the table so that it could be dealt with at the outset as an issue in the psychotherapy.

The Therapeutic Frame

The wish for mothering or fathering is one example of a broader issue that makes optimal distance difficult to establish in the beginning of a psychotherapy process with borderline patients. Almost all the usual boundaries of treatment—which constitute the therapeutic frame—are challenged or tested by the patient. In the vignette featuring Ms. Y, the patient wished to establish the therapeutic frame on her own terms instead of the therapist's terms. Matters such as frequency and duration of sessions, phone calls between hours, length of sessions, and professional forms of address are usually established by the therapist according to guidelines of professional conduct. However, Ms. Y suggested that she would require four sessions a week (as opposed to the two suggested by Dr. B); she suggested that she should be allowed up to 10 phone calls per week to deal with crises; she asked if she could address her therapist by her first name; and she made it quite clear that she would have difficulty leaving after the 50-minute session.

Other patients may request special fee arrangements, including no payment at all, extratherapeutic contacts, and physical touch as part of the process. The therapeutic frame is like an envelope or membrane around the therapeutic role that defines the characteristics of the therapeutic relationship (Langs 1976; Spruiell 1983). The elements of the frame are constructed out of the various parameters of treatment, including frequency and duration of appointments, absence of physical contact, specific forms of appropriate social behavior, language, mode of dress, fee arrangements, and the office setting itself (Gutheil and Gabbard 1993). These boundaries function as limits that maintain the optimal psychotherapeutic distance in the relationship so that both parties can enter a symbolic realm where ideas can be examined in a collaborative way by patient and therapist.

One of the most useful ways to manage countertransference reactions and establish optimal distance is to clarify the treatment boundaries at the beginning of a psychotherapeutic process. In the case of Ms. Y, for example, the therapist clearly will need to spend some time helping the patient understand what are realistic expectations of a therapeutic relationship and what are unrealistic false hopes that will lead to disillusionment. Among the common countertransference problems in the psychotherapy of borderline patients is that therapists begin to believe they actually may be better parents than the real parents. They may feel coerced into a parental role as though no other interaction will be of any use whatsoever. The decision to attempt to "out-mother" the patient's actual mother is doomed to failure from the outset because a therapeutic relationship can never provide what a parental relationship provides in reality. As Spruiell (1983) noted, "it is as disastrous for analysts to actually treat their patients like children as it is for analysts to treat their own children as patients" (p. 12).

Kernberg and colleagues (1989) wrote eloquently on the establishment of an initial contractual understanding with the patient that serves the purpose of educating the patient about realistic expectations for the therapeutic process while at the same time informing the patient implicitly that therapists have rights and will not submit themselves to abuse. Before therapists agree to start a psychotherapy process, they must have an agreement from the patient that the treatment structure will be followed. For example, matters such as the fee payment, the length of sessions, the handling of vacations, the frequency of sessions, the need for psychiatric hospitalization, the management of suicidal crises, and a general understanding about phone calls between sessions can all be laid out as part of the initial contract. Establishing these boundaries or parameters of the treatment also serves as a valuable adjunct in managing countertransference. Any deviation from the standard therapeutic frame can alert the therapist to the emergence of countertransference reactions.

Some borderline patients will present a good deal of reluctance when asked to agree to the structure of the treatment. Therapists must be prepared to come to the conclusion that no psychotherapeutic work will be possible if the patient is unable to agree to the treatment conditions (Kernberg et al. 1989). Therapists of borderline patients must always remind themselves that there are much worse fates than termination of the treatment. It is better not to begin at all than to begin under grossly misguided circumstances.

One of the most effective ways to maintain the appropriate professional distance in the early going is to make the therapeutic frame the main focus of the sessions. It is helpful to remind the patient continually that psychotherapy has not yet begun. Until the negotiations are successfully completed regarding the treatment structure, the process is basically a consultation or evaluation. Therapists can also use this opportunity to delineate the patient's responsibility for collaborating in a psychological, exploratory process. Fantasies of being passively healed by a perfect parent can be brought up from the beginning and addressed as unrealistic. A successfully negotiated initial contract may be one of the best prophylactic measures involved in the successful management of countertransference later in the treatment.

Another reason for the special attention to establishing a contract during the initial period is that the therapeutic frame contributes to the formation of the therapeutic alliance. Best defined as a mutual collaboration between patient and therapist in pursuit of common therapeutic goals, the therapeutic alliance is a critical ingredient in the success of psychotherapy with borderline patients (Gabbard et al. 1988; Meissner 1988). Patients who make a sincere commitment to the contractual understanding are implicitly agreeing to a perspective that involves forming a collaborative working relationship.

Countertransference Rigidity
Rationalized as Textbook Technique

One of the paradoxes in psychotherapy of borderline patients is that the practice of setting the structure for the treatment may itself become a fertile field for countertransference enactment. Many beginning therapists (and even more seasoned ones) respond to their anxiety about the patient's near-magnetic pull to transgress the therapeutic frame by becoming excessively rigid. The term *borderline* is often used pejoratively as a synonym for "manipulator," "splitter," or "pain in the neck." The patient's transference wishes to be mothered may be regarded as a malevolent assault on the therapist's professional competence and integrity. This countertransference perception may be handled by assuming a steely, withholding posture so as not to be "taken in" by the patient. Such strategies may then be rationalized as textbook technique—an example of "setting firm limits."

Another way to understand the therapist's withdrawal and attitude of nonresponsiveness is that they are directly proportional to the perceived object hunger and affective intensity of the patient. Therapists may feel that they are being drawn into a maelstrom of affect where they, too, will undergo a merger that involves a loss of self. As Lewin and Schulz (1992) observed, "the therapist presents the patient with a threat of loss in order to protect against what he sees as a dangerous invitation to fusion" (p. 80). In this countertransference distancing maneuver, the therapist is behaving as though the patient's all-or-none point of view is an unalterable reality that must be contended with. The therapist is inadvertently "buying in" to the notion that no middle ground exists. Throughout the psychotherapy process with borderline patients, therapists must repeatedly strive to find a reasonable middle ground in the context of the patient's coercion to view the situation as an either/or choice between catastrophic polarities.

Virtually every session of psychotherapy with a borderline patient involves a countertransference dilemma regarding the extent to which partial gratification of transference wishes is indicated. The therapist must decide which is the greater technical error: complete deprivation or partial gratification? A judgment call must be made in such circumstances based on the therapist's best assessment at the time. One helpful guideline is the distinction drawn by Casement (1985) between "libidinal demands" and "growth needs." The former cannot be gratified without gravely jeopardizing the treatment and committing serious ethical compromises. The latter cannot be frustrated without preventing growth. Casement's notion of growth needs can be understood as what has traditionally been termed the provision of *a holding environment.*

Consistency is, to be sure, an essential aspect of the holding environment. But as Casement (1990) noted, "paradoxically, a part of the consistency that a patient needs from the analyst is that of *empathic responsiveness to changing needs,* which means the analyst sometimes adapting to the patient rather than remaining rigidly the same" (p. 333). A patient, for example, may need the therapist to take a more active stance regarding verbal interventions because of experiencing silence as a retraumatization that parallels childhood experiences with a cold, withholding mother. Another patient may need to make a brief phone call to the therapist over a long weekend because of a severe lack of object constancy. A few words from the therapist may immediately restore the therapist as an alive and vital presence for the patient and put to rest the catastrophic anxiety that had arisen during the separation.

These partial transference gratifications may serve to create an atmosphere that makes psychotherapy possible. Certain growth needs must be met, or there may be no treatment at all. The degree to which these needs are met has a great deal to do with the location of the therapist's technique on the expressive-supportive continuum. Therapists must base their decisions regarding technique on a careful assessment of patient characteristics (Gabbard 1994; Meissner 1988). Even the partial gratifications that occur in supportive therapy, however, are still ultimately disappointing because they fall short of the patient's longings for unconditional "mother love." Moreover, supportive interventions that may be gratifying to the patient must be geared specifically to the patients' areas of weakened ego functioning. Rockland (1992), who developed a systematic approach to supportive psychotherapy for borderline patients, issued the following cautionary statement:

> It is in the supportive psychotherapy of the [borderline personality disorder] patient that the therapist's ability to utilize countertransference reactions without acting them out, that is, to use support, advice, praise, or limit setting *only as required by the patient's ego deficits,* and not to gratify conscious or unconscious wishes of the therapist, receives its most challenging test. (p. 190)

Acknowledging the need for flexibility, however, should not minimize the necessity of boundaries. Some transference wishes—such as wanting to be physically held—should not be gratified under any circumstances. For one thing, from a risk-management perspective, therapists who hug their patients are skating on thin ice (Gutheil and Gabbard 1993). Moreover, from a strictly clinical perspective, literally holding the patient collapses the analytic space and blurs the distinction between the symbolic and the concrete (Casement 1990). Finally, such an act may provide the patient with false hope that the therapist really will become the parent so earnestly desired.

The therapist must ultimately fail the patient. Only through failing to meet the patient's all-consuming needs will the necessary disillusionment and mourning process take hold in psychotherapy. Attempting to be the "all-good" mother is doomed to failure. The role is not only impossible to sustain but is inherently nontherapeutic. Patients need to experience the therapist as the "old object" from childhood to work through the vicissitudes of the internal object relationships that emerge in the transference. This necessary therapeutic work is bypassed when therapists represent themselves as perfect objects, suggesting that saintly persons are available if the patient can only locate them.

The oscillation between the new object and the old object is instrumental to successful psychotherapy of borderline patients. In this regard, Greenberg's (1986) contemporary definition of neutrality is germane. In his view, neutrality "embodies the goal of establishing an optimal tension between the patient's tendency to see the analyst as an old object and his capacity to experience him as a new one" (p. 97). This reconceptualization of the time-honored psychoanalytic concept allows for much greater flexibility by therapists and is therefore a more suitable definition for their stance vis-à-vis the borderline patient. An absolutely nonjudgmental role that is equidistant from ego, id, and superego might be actively harmful in treating many borderline patients who have suffered from parental neglect, abuse, or indifference. Patients must be actively confronted if their behavior is self-destructive or threatens to destroy the therapist or the treatment itself (Waldinger 1987).

Greenberg's definition also captures the ebb and flow of transference-countertransference enactments followed by a systematic processing of those enactments that characterize the day-in–day-out drama of psychotherapy with borderline patients. Through the process of projective identification, therapists find themselves in the obligatory role of "the heavy" one day, and "the saint" the next, before they finally return to some semblance of their familiar professional persona. One soon learns that neither the persecuting bad object nor the idealized all-good object is in itself therapeutic. Only the new "real" object of the therapist (as a consistent figure who reflects on the experiences within the dyad that lead to the coerced old object experiences) leads to significant change. A reasonable goal for a borderline patient's therapist is to be a "not-bad" object. After all, most of us would be content if all our family members and friends could simply meet this compromise between ideals and reality.

Summary

From the first contact between therapist and patient, establishing optimal distance is a high priority. Borderline patients repeatedly test the professional boundaries of the relationship and often directly or indirectly express a wish for a parent rather than a therapist. Early in the psychotherapy process, the therapist often feels a sense of floundering and an inner urgency to act rather than reflect. Because of the potential for pharmacotherapy to be contaminated by countertransference responses, a rational and systematic approach to medication, based on target symptoms and trait vulnerabilities, must be part of the overall treatment plan. Establishing a therapeutic frame and a contractual understanding is a useful way to construct an analytic space with the patient in which psychotherapy can take place. Matters such as fee payment, the length of sessions, the handling of vacations, the frequency of sessions, the need for psychiatric hospitalization, the management of suicidal crises, and a policy on phone calls should be part of this contract. On the other hand, a good deal of countertransference enactment can hide behind the rigid adherence to an inflexible structure. The balance between flexibility and boundaries parallels the therapist's oscillation between playing the role of a new object in the present and an old object from the past.

References

Bollas C: The Shadow of the Object: Psychoanalysis of the Unthought Known. New York, Columbia University Press, 1987

Casement P: On Learning From the Patient. London, Tavistock, 1985

Casement PJ: The meeting of the needs in psychoanalysis. Psychoanalytic Inquiry 10:325–346, 1990

Cowdry RW, Gardner DL: Pharmacotherapy of borderline personality disorder: alprazolam, carbamazepine, trifluoperazine, and tranylcypromine. Arch Gen Psychiatry 45:111–119, 1988

Gabbard GO: Psychodynamic Psychiatry in Clinical Practice: The DSM-IV Edition. Washington, DC, American Psychiatric Press, 1994

Gabbard GO, Horwitz L, Frieswyk S, et al: The effect of therapist interventions on the therapeutic alliance with borderline patients. J Am Psychoanal Assoc 36:697–727, 1988

Greenberg JR: Theoretical models and the analyst's neutrality. Contemporary Psychoanalysis 22:87–106, 1986

Gutheil TG, Gabbard GO: The concept of boundaries in clinical practice: theoretical and risk management dimensions. Am J Psychiatry 150:188–196, 1993

Kernberg OF, Selzer MA, Koenigsberg HW, et al: Psychodynamic Psychotherapy of Borderline Patients. New York, Basic Books, 1989

Langs R: The Bipersonal Field. New York, Jason Aronson, 1976

Lewin RA, Schulz CG: Losing and Fusing: Borderline and Transitional Object and Self Relations. Northvale, NJ, Jason Aronson, 1992

Meissner WW: Treatment of Patients in the Borderline Spectrum. Northvale, NJ, Jason Aronson, 1988

Ogden TH: The Matrix of the Mind: Object Relations and the Psychoanalytic Dialogue. Northvale, NJ, Jason Aronson, 1986

Rockland LH: Supportive Therapy for Borderline Patients: A Psychodynamic Approach. New York, Guilford, 1992

Soloff PH: Pharmacological therapies in borderline personality disorder, in Borderline Personality Disorder: Etiology and Treatment. Edited by Paris J. Washington, DC, American Psychiatric Press, 1993, pp 319–348

Spruiell V: The rules and frames of the psychoanalytic situation. Psychoanal Q 52:1–33, 1983

Waldinger RJ: Intensive psychodynamic therapy with borderline patients: an overview. Am J Psychiatry 144:267–274, 1987

Waldinger RJ, Frank AF: Clinicians' experiences in combining medication and psychotherapy in the treatment of borderline patients. Hosp Community Psychiatry 40:712–718, 1989

CHAPTER 3

On Victims, Rescuers, and Abusers

One of the most powerful sources of countertransference difficulties in the psychotherapy of borderline patients is the perception of the patient as a victim. Neurotic patients seem to make more of an authorial contribution to their sagas of misery and unhappiness. They seem to be unfair and unforgiving toward their parents, and the role of their own distortions and fantasies in their interpersonal problems is apparent.

With borderline patients, on the other hand, one often hears heart-rending stories of cruel abuse and neglect at the hands of caregivers. A compelling feature of such stories is the patient's profound helplessness as a child being dealt a cruel hand by fate. Many of the patients themselves, despite having been subjected to mistreatment by others, steadfastly blame themselves with the assumption that they must basically be bad persons to have been treated in such a manner. All of these factors taken together are likely to evoke rescue fantasies in treaters. Therapists often find themselves thinking inwardly, "if only this engaging and bright young person had had different parents, things would be so different," or "if only this unfortunate woman would meet the right man who would not treat her like these other men did." Such internal musings often reflect a nascent rescue fantasy involving the therapist as perfect parent or perfect lover who will snatch the patient from the jaws of fate and magically transform the patient's life.

Recent empirical research has largely substantiated the notion that many borderline patients have experienced real victimization in their childhood relationships with parents and other caretakers. In contrast to some of the psychodynamic theories of pathogenesis that stress excessive constitutional aggression (Kernberg 1975) or maternal overinvolvement (Masterson and Rinsley 1975), empirical research over the last two decades suggests that frank physical and sexual abuse and gross neglect play a key role in the etiology of borderline personality disorder, at least in certain cases. A family study of borderline patients (Walsh 1977) found that 64% of the probands reported highly conflicted relationships with their parents, characterized by frank abuse, parental hostility, and overt devaluation.

Since Walsh's (1977) original study, numerous reports have confirmed a high incidence of abuse during childhood in the history of borderline patients. Herman and colleagues (1989) found that 68% of a sample of 21 borderline patients had been sexually abused as children, 71% had been physically abused, and 62% had witnessed serious domestic violence. Westen and colleagues (1990) were able to find evidence of physical or sexual abuse in more than 50% of the medical records of inpatient adolescents diagnosed with borderline personality disorder.

Ogata and colleagues (1990) compared experiences of abuse and neglect in 24 borderline adults with those of 18 depressed control subjects. In the borderline group, 71% had a history of childhood sexual abuse, 10% had a history of physical abuse, 17% reported a history of physical neglect, and 65% reported multiple abuses. When compared with the control group of depressed patients, the incidence of childhood sexual abuse and combined sexual and physical abuse was significantly higher for the borderline patients. No differences were found between groups for either neglect or physical abuse unaccompanied by sexual abuse.

Another comparison study (Zanarini et al. 1989) categorized childhood abuse in one of three forms: verbal, physical, and sexual. The investigators compared 50 borderline outpatients with 26 outpatients who had dysthymia and 29 who had antisocial personality disorder. Of the borderline patients, 58% reported a history of sexual abuse, physical abuse, or both. Verbal abuse, however, was actually more common than either physical or sexual abuse. Fully 72%

of the borderline patients reported verbal abuse as compared with 46% with physical abuse and 26% with sexual abuse. In the same sample, 76% reported significant neglect by parents or caretakers during childhood.

Baker and colleagues (1992) studied 29 borderline inpatients compared with 15 depressive patients and 14 nonpsychiatric control subjects. Borderline patients rated their parents, especially their fathers, not only as more unfavorable on negative scales than control subjects and depressive patients but as less favorable on positive scales than the comparison groups. A significant portion of the variance in father scores, but not in mother scores, was related to the age of the respondent and the history of sexual abuse. The investigators concluded that these borderline patients had a greater tendency to view the world in negative, malevolent ways than the patients in the comparison groups. Also, 77.4% of the borderline patients reported histories of sexual abuse compared with only 33% of the depressed patients and 21.4% of the control group. However, only 35.5% of the borderline patients had experienced incestuous sexual abuse, with 16.1% reporting abuse by the father, 3.2% abuse by the mother, and 25.8% abuse by siblings.

Zanarini and colleagues (1989) also studied the separation histories of the borderline patients and control subjects, and 74% had experienced loss or prolonged separation from a caretaker during some period before age 18. This finding, although striking, was not too dissimilar from that found in antisocial patients and dysthymic patients. However, when the separations were examined for the period of early childhood, borderline patients had a significantly higher percentage than did dysthymic patients.

At least five major studies (Frank and Paris 1981; Goldberg et al. 1985; Paris and Frank 1989; Soloff and Millward 1983; Zweig-Frank and Paris 1991) suggest that borderline patients experience their parents as emotionally neglectful. In the most recent of these studies (Zweig-Frank and Paris 1991), 62 borderline patients were compared with 99 nonborderline patients through the use of the Parental Bonding Instrument. As might be expected, borderline patients were significantly more likely to remember their fathers and mothers as having been less caring than the control group. Although many of the psychodynamic theories focus on maternal failures in the etiology and pathogenesis of borderline pathology, this study indicated that *both parents* are remembered as creating difficulties during the childhoods of these patients. There was a pattern of "affectionless control" in that both parents failed to provide emotional support *and* prevented the children from separating. Zweig-Frank and Paris referred to this pattern as "bi-parental failure" and pointed out that borderline patients as children were unable to have their negative experiences with one parent buffered by more positive experiences with the other parent.

The results of all these empirical investigations taken together suggest a mixed and complex picture of the etiology and pathogenesis of borderline personality disorder. Clearly, there are many pathways to the development of borderline psychopathology. Many patients have experienced some combination of loss, neglect, physical abuse, verbal abuse, and sexual abuse. Some of the contradictory views expressed in the psychodynamic theories may stem from differing developmental experiences in different populations of borderline patients (Gabbard 1994). For example, patients who have experienced early childhood loss or neglect may fail to develop a holding-soothing introject, as described by Adler (1985). The work of Zweig-Frank and Paris (1991) indicates that other patients experienced overcontrol in childhood (by both mother and father) and therefore may experience abandonment concerns such as those described by Masterson and Rinsley (1975).

In each study a subgroup of borderline patients without a history of abuse and neglect could possibly fit Kernberg's (1975) model of excessive constitutional aggression. Clinicians must be wary of a knee-jerk readiness to blame parents for all the difficulties that accompany borderline personality disorder. One inpatient, for example, reported that during the Cuban missile crisis in the early 1960s, her mother said she would murder the patient in her bed so that she would not have to endure a nuclear war. When the social worker met with the mother, who appeared to be a genuinely concerned and caring person, she was aghast to hear that her daughter had distorted so greatly what had happened. The patient's mother clarified that she had made a comment to the effect that the family might be better off dead than to have to suffer the effects of an atomic blast.

Countertransference Reactions to the Patient as Victim

The therapist's perception of the patient as a victim—a perception that may be entirely valid in reality—results in specific forms of therapeutic zeal that may ultimately be counterproductive. In many cases therapists are characterologically predisposed to rescue fantasies because of childhood constellations involving a depressed mother or father and a long-standing pattern of playing the role of therapist in the family (Gabbard, in press; Sussman 1992). Hence the rescuer role, evoked through projective identification by the patient's self-presentation as a victim, may attach to the therapist's preexisting internal need to be a rescuer, and the two elements may function synergistically to produce formidable countertransference enactments.

One of the most striking examples of the countertransference consequences of seeing the patient as a victim can be found by studying the clinical diary of Sandor Ferenczi (Dupont 1988). Disillusioned with his analytic experience with Freud, Ferenczi adopted a new technique to deal with female patients whom he viewed as victims of actual sexual trauma during childhood. He differed with Freud's emphasis on the role of fantasy and felt that these patients needed to be loved because of the absence of love as a child.

Ferenczi called his method the "relaxation technique" and geared it to the creation of a safe atmosphere in which the patient's longings could be gratified by the analyst without making any demands (Hoffer 1991). In his view he was re-creating the early symbiotic bliss of the mother-infant relationship.

Many psychotherapists harbor a conscious or unconscious fantasy that love in and of itself may be curative (Gabbard, in press). Ferenczi grew up in a family in which his mother was so busy with other siblings that she was unable to provide her son with the kind of emotional nurturance that he felt he required (Grubrich-Simitis 1986). As a result Ferenczi longed to be loved, and his therapeutic efforts can be understood as a way of trying to provide for his patients what he himself did not receive as a child. Similarly, in this confusion of his own needs and his patients' needs, he may have secretly hoped to be loved and idealized in return for his loving, therapeutic efforts.

A detailed examination of Ferenczi's diary entries suggests, however, that his efforts to love his patients was a reaction formation to intense feelings of hatred and aggression (Gabbard 1992). In one diary entry on May 5, 1932, Ferenczi noted: "The patient's demands to be loved corresponded to analogous demands on me by my mother. In actual fact and inwardly, therefore, I did hate the patient, in spite of all the friendliness I displayed" (Dupont 1988, p. 99). Ferenczi had grown up harboring tremendous resentment toward his mother, and he recognized in this entry that childhood feelings of hatred toward her had been displaced onto his patient. One can speculate that Ferenczi's efforts to be like "an affectionate mother" with his patients was not only designed to give them the love that he had himself missed in childhood, but also an unconscious attempt to repair damage he felt he had inflicted on his own mother. This historical example beautifully illustrates the process of mutual projective identification. While his incest-victim patients were projecting an idealized rescuer introject into Ferenczi, he was alternately projecting his own child-victim self-representation and his hated-mother object-representation into the patients.

Two extremes on the countertransference continuum are common in response to incest victims. Ferenczi's attempts to provide a reparenting experience for his patients is emblematic of one extreme—overidentification with the victim combined with zealous rescue fantasies. This response is also characterized by the view that incest explains all the patient's psychopathology. On the opposite end of the continuum is a reaction of skepticism or frank disbelief. Many clinicians still do not believe the reports of victimization voiced by their patients. They may unwittingly retraumatize their patients by functioning as a jurist engaged in a process of determining evidence and proof rather than as a therapist attempting to understand. In this manner they may be reenacting a childhood situation in which the patient tried to explain to an adult what was going on, only to be disbelieved.

From a psychotherapeutic perspective, a more rational and clinically useful position is to steer a middle course between the two extremes. Therapists can empathize with the psychic reality of the trauma in their patients without assuming that every detail is historically correct. Adult borderline patients rarely fabricate extensive childhood trauma, even though a particular event may be distorted in one way or anther when recalled. Moreover, the pathogenic nature of traumatic childhood experiences can be validated without having to abandon the conceptual framework that multiple etiologic factors converge to produce borderline personality disorder, one of which is childhood trauma.

An Unfolding Drama

The example of Ferenczi illustrates a pattern that can most usefully be understood as an unfolding drama involving four principal characters: a victim, an abuser, an idealized and omnipotent rescuer, and an uninvolved mother (Davies and Frawley 1992; Gabbard 1992). These characters oscillate in various complementary pairings between patient and therapist through the transference-countertransference enactments that develop in the psychotherapy. Although originally described in a dialogue regarding the treatment of incest victims, they apply more generally to the psychotherapy of borderline patients who have been victimized in other ways as well.

The first three characters in the dramatis personae—the victim, the abuser, and the idealized and omnipotent rescuer—unfold in a predictable pattern that represents a convergence of countertransference in the narrow sense with countertransference in the broad sense via projective identification. When a history of victimization or childhood abuse emerges in the patient, something powerful tugs on the heartstrings of therapists that urges them to become a better parent than the ones who victimized the patient. As was the case with Ferenczi, this role-responsive reaction to the patient often attaches itself to preexisting wishes to rescue or repair objects from the therapist's past.

This rescuer-victim paradigm with which the psychotherapy begins, however, is fraught with problems. The patient is not likely to see the therapist's motives in the same way the therapist sees them. Patients who have been abused as children often assume that everyone will abuse them because they have no reason to think otherwise. As a way of making sense out of a seemingly senseless universe, these children assume that they must have deserved the abuse they received. This point of view allows such patients to salvage a view of their parents as abusing them out of love and concern rather than a more horrifying possibility—that the violence against them was a random product of a malevolent universe.

Given this perspective, these patients are inherently mistrustful of reassurances from therapists who assert that they will not abuse the patient. Moreover, therapists who reassure such patients that they were *not* responsible for what happened in the patients' childhood are not likely to get very far with that approach. The patients will simply feel that the therapist does not understand the situation. Reassurances may make therapists feel better, but they rarely make patients feel better. Professions of caring are intrinsically suspect to patients who have been exploited under the guise of being loved.

Patients who have been victims of sexual abuse do not have the benefit of growing up with generational boundaries and limits enforced by effective, caring parents. They often experience the professional boundaries of the therapeutic situation as a cruel form of withholding. They may demand demonstrations of caring that involve extended sessions, physical contact, self-disclosure from the therapist, and round-the-clock availability. If therapists begin to "run the extra mile" to gratify these requests, their efforts are doomed to failure. As noted in Chapter 2, the attempt to become a parental substitute bypasses the patient's need to mourn and raises false hopes that a parental relationship is available if only the patient can find the right person.

Another possible determinant of such ill-advised efforts to rescue the patient may be the therapist's underlying feelings of despair after hearing a frank confession from the patient about a history of incest or other sexual abuse. Often this confession is presented with a certain degree of finality, suggesting that the sexual abuse is the unquestionable source of all the patient's problems and should be taken at face value. On hearing a patient acknowledge sexual abuse, Bollas (1989) described a sinking feeling that has to do with the fantasy that he has lost the right to analyze in response to the patient's loss of reflective thought. This feeling is intimately related to the collapse of analytic space in patients who are incest victims. When the father sexually violates his daughter, that child no longer has the option of fantasy about the father as her knight in shining armor. The transitional realm of play has been decimated. This collapse of transitional or analytic space makes it difficult for such patients to maintain the "as if" quality of the transference (Levine 1990). Fantasies about the therapist are taken as realities, not as symbolic constructs to be analyzed.

When therapists attempt to gratify the patient's escalating demands for evidence that the therapist cares, the patient's sense of entitlement is activated. Treatment of sexually abused borderline patients sooner or later reveals an underlying conviction that they are entitled to compensation in the present for the abuse they have experienced in the past (Davies and Frawley 1992). As the demands further escalate, the therapist may soon develop a feeling of being tormented. Through processes of introjective and projective identification, the characters in the dramatis personae have changed in such a way that the therapist has become the victim and the patient has become an abuser. Clinicians who treat borderline patients with a history of childhood abuse must never forget that an abusive parent has been internalized and thus exists as an introject ready to be activated at the drop of a hat. In this regard, a study by Nigg and colleagues (1991) is particularly relevant. These investigators studied 29 borderline inpatients in comparison with 15 nonpsychiatric control subjects and 14 depressed patients. A clear linkage was found between extremely malevolent object-representations in the earliest memories of the borderline patients and a history of sexual abuse. Childhood physical abuse did *not* predict the presence of such introjects. Similarly, borderline patients who lacked a history of sexual abuse did not show signs of such malevolent object-representations. The researchers noted that these patients expect abuse in psychotherapy while also hoping for a benevolent protector to disconfirm their expectations.

At any rate, abusive or malevolent introjects residing within the patient may take hold of the patient while the victim-self of the patient is projected into the therapist. Moreover, therapists may create a fertile field for this identification with the patient-victim self-representation as a result of their guilt feelings related to the growing resentment and hatred toward the patient. Patients may sense this development and accuse the therapist of not really caring. In an effort to deny the feeling of resentment at being asked to do too much and to go too far, therapists try even harder to prove that their motives are pure. At such moments therapists may secretly feel that they have been "found out" and react by trying to mask their irritation. An acknowledgment of limits may be the most therapeutic way to manage one's countertransference feelings when things reach this point. The following clinical vignette (Gabbard 1986) illustrates the unfolding drama that we have just described:

> Ms. X was a 24-year-old woman who had a history of a 10-year-long sexual relationship with her father. She came to a psychiatric hospital 3 years after the incestuous relationship had stopped because of chronic suicidal and self-mutilating behavior. The incestuous involvement had come to a halt when she had told her mother about it. Her mother's reaction was to fly into a rage at Ms. X for having "an affair" with her father. Her mother told her that she never wanted to speak to her again.
>
> At the time of her admission, Ms. X told Dr. C a poignant history of having been repeatedly abused by her father and rejected by her mother. Despite her horrendous past, she managed to maintain some sense of humor and was able to charm Dr. C with her engaging smile and her wish to change her condition so she could get on with her life. Dr. C immediately felt a powerful wish to demonstrate to her that men could be trusted and could care about her without violating her.
>
> In the initial interviews with Dr. C, Ms. X made a request. She

said that she had never talked with anyone about the details of her incestuous relationship with her father. She felt intense shame about these sexual acts and told Dr. C that she could only discuss them with him if he would make an exception to his usual practice of sharing the contents of his interviews with the rest of the hospital treatment team. After reflecting a moment, Dr. C acceded to Ms. X's request. He was aware that he was making an exception to the usual practice of sharing information freely with staff, but he rationalized the exception by arguing to himself that if he were to violate Ms. X's request, he would simply be repeating her history of exploitation by parading her unfortunate and sordid history in front of a voyeuristic audience of prurient staff members.

As Ms. X began to reveal a horrific history involving 10 years of perverse sexual acts with her father, Dr. C was deeply shocked and found himself enraged at Ms. X's father. He began to develop a formulation regarding the patient's self-mutilation and suicidal wishes. Eventually Dr. C interpreted to the patient that her self-mutilation was a way of punishing herself for participation in the incestuous relationship with her father and expressing her rage at him for exploiting her. When Dr. C offered this intervention, Ms. X looked at him in a quizzical way as though his comment made no sense whatsoever to her. She explained to him that, in fact, her father had made her feel special and loved, in contrast to her mother, whom Ms. X felt was rejecting and harsh. She went on to elaborate that her depression and suicidal behavior had been brought on by the *cessation* of the sexual relationship with her father.

Dr. C found himself almost imperceptibly recoiling from Ms. X's clarification of her experience. He realized that he had imposed his own feelings of loathing and disgust for the father onto Ms. X. The patient had become a container for his own feelings. As a result, he was not as receptive as he might have been to listening to her own experience and validating it as different from his own. His wish to rescue Ms. X from her history of abuse at the hands of others had become a powerful therapeutic mission that had led him to deviate from his usual way of working in hospital treatment and caused him to engage in a countertransference enactment. In his misinterpretation of the patient's self-mutilation, he was revealing his own rage at the father and his sense of competitiveness born of his wish to be a better father.

The rescuer-victim paradigm in the transference-countertransference relationship between Dr. C and Ms. X followed the predictable path of evolving into a victim-abuser relationship when the patient became intensely suicidal during her hospital stay. One night as Dr. C was leaving the hospital, Ms. X told him that she felt like killing herself. In the same breath she admonished Dr. C not to increase the structure around her by locking the door and putting her on suicide watchfulness. When Dr. C asked Ms. X if she could talk to staff before acting on her wish to leave the hospital and kill herself, she said she thought she could but was hesitant in her response. Dr. C told her that he would arrange to have special nurses watch her during the night because of her uncertainty about her controls. Ms. X reacted with an accusatory stare and an air of contempt: "You don't listen to what I say, do you? You do what *you* think I need rather than what I tell you I need."

Dr. C responded strongly to Ms. X's accusations. Indeed, he had misinterpreted her self-mutilation in the past out of his own need to see her difficulties in a particular manner, growing out of his own countertransference reactions. He decided to trust her in the midst of this crisis situation in hopes that a more durable therapeutic alliance would result from his trust. He left the hospital without changing her level of restriction, even though it was against his better judgment.

Later that night he received a phone call informing him that Ms. X had left the hospital. He felt betrayed by her, as though she had made a fool of him. When she returned to the hospital after an episode of mutilation, Dr. C went in to see Ms. X. She refused to talk to him and treated him with a remote, contemptuous attitude, as though he were of no significance in her life.

In the ensuing days, the patient was intensely suicidal and repeatedly struggled with overwhelming urges to kill herself in the middle of the night. Typically, around 2 or 3 A.M., Ms. X would tell the nurses on her unit that she was about to kill herself and needed restraints to keep her from acting on it. The nurses would call Dr. C at home and ask him for a restraint order. Each night Dr. C was awakened to give the order and then found himself lying in bed awake as he contemplated whether he was doing the right thing.

This nightly pattern of being awakened in the middle of the night took its toll. Dr. C felt that he was not functioning as well as he should during the day, and each night he dreaded going to sleep because he knew he would be awakened. He was aware that he felt tormented by Ms. X and realized that he had now become the victim of the abusive introject within her. He said to her that he now realized what it was like to be her. He also told her that he wondered if she were so insecure about the capacity of others to care for her that she felt she had to constantly test her treaters. Ms. X acknowledged anxiety about her treaters' capacity to care and confided a deep fear of abandonment to Dr. C. In the context of this conversation, Dr. C told her that he could not function during the day if he continued to be awakened each night dealing with her suicidal crises. He further explained to her that he had limits that were now being exceeded. He did not wish to abandon her, he explained, but he would not be able to continue meeting these nightly demands for attention.

This combination of acknowledging his limits and helping the patient to clarify her underlying abandonment fear led to a major breakthrough in the treatment. Ms. X no longer required restraints in the middle of the night, and Dr. C no longer felt tormented.

Although this cautionary tale illustrates the first two acts in the unfolding drama—therapist as rescuer in response to patient as victim leading to therapist as victim in response to patient as abuser— it does not depict the third act of the drama. In certain instances when the escalating pattern of increasing demands by the patient is accompanied by increasing efforts to gratify those demands by the therapist, a third transference-countertransference paradigm may emerge. At the height of exasperation with the failing of all therapeutic efforts, therapists may resort to drastic boundary crossings with the patient that in effect repeat the childhood abuse. The therapist has become the abuser with the patient once again in the role of victim. The most tragic and all-too-common manifestation of this third paradigm is overt sexual contact between therapist and patient. Other common examples include sadistic verbal abuse of the patient, attempts to provide nurturance by sitting the patient on one's lap and "reparenting" the patient, taking the patient on family outings with the therapist's family, and so forth. In such situations the therapist's rage at being thwarted is often completely disavowed. What began as a rescue effort has ended up as a reenactment of exploitation and abuse.

Many victims of childhood sexual abuse suffer from a form of learned helplessness where they feel that no effort on their part can change their fate. They believe that when one is trapped, there is no recourse. These patients have no sense of agency or efficacy to call on. In this sense they are "sitting ducks" (Kluft 1989) for all forms of abuse and boundary violations by therapists who are using their patients to gratify their own needs.

The Uninvolved Mother

The three roles of victim, abuser, and idealized and omnipotent rescuer are the most dramatic and obvious manifestations of the introjective-projective processes at work in the psychotherapy of borderline patients. The fourth role, the uninvolved mother, occurs in a somewhat more subtle way. Patients will often perceive this figure in the therapist's silence, which is interpreted as indifference and rejection. In response to this perception of indifference, the patient may feel a sense of nonbeing, described by Bigras and Biggs (1990) as "negative incest," a deadness or emptiness related to the absent mother who made no attempt to intervene in the incestuous relationship between her husband and daughter.

The deadness or emptiness experienced by the patient may foster complementary feelings of helplessness and despair in the psychotherapist. There may be long periods in the psychotherapy of borderline patients with a history of incest where the patient remains aloof and distant from the therapist and evokes feelings of deadness or nonbeing in the countertransference (Levine 1990; Lisman-Pieczanski 1990).

Countertransference responses of this nature may reflect an empathic identification with the nonbeing at the core of the patient's self in response to the distant maternal identification in the patient. There also comes a time in the psychotherapy of borderline patients who have been sexually abused where the demandingness of the patient is so overwhelming that therapists find themselves wishing the patient would disappear or go else-where for treatment. In such reactions it is not difficult to detect an identification with the uninvolved mother, and therapists must be mindful that such unconscious collusions may lead unwittingly to suicide attempts.

The primitive states of psychological deadness depicted in this transference-countertransference paradigm may relate to pro-found maternal deprivation that severely compromises the infant's developing sense of self. In the absence of maternal provision of soothing sensory experience, the infant may not establish a secure feeling of sensory boundedness. The self-mutilation so common in borderline patients with a history of sexual abuse (who may also have dissociative disorders) can be understood as a way of reestab-lishing boundedness at the skin border to deal with anxiety about losing intactness of the ego boundary. Ogden (1989) characterized this mode of generating experience as the autistic-contiguous posi-tion. In this primitive state there is a cessation of the process of attributing meaning to experience. Therapists may experience bor-derline patients imprisoned in such a primitive state as completely unreachable and therefore may be imbued with a sense of hopeless-ness in dealing with the patient's anxiety about lack of body integ-rity based on deprivation from close sensory experiences with mother.

Countertransference Responses to Suicidality

The relentless suicidality and self-destructive behavior of many bor-derline patients often inspire extraordinary rescue fantasies in ther-apists. Although many patients make repeated gestures without seriously intending to kill themselves, longitudinal follow-up stud-ies suggest that the suicide rate among borderline patients may be as high as 8% (Stone 1990). Besides stoking the fires of omnipo-tence in the therapist, suicidality may also be a source of torment. Patients often wield suicidal threats like the Sword of Damocles held over the therapist's head. If the therapist does not do the patient's bidding, or if the therapist does not say exactly the right words, the patient will retaliate with a suicide attempt.

When patients discern that the therapist is anxious about their potential to commit suicide, they may then exploit the therapist's anxiety. For example, some therapists will talk more, offer more support, and gratify more transference wishes whenever the patient talks of suicide. The astute patient will soon learn that bringing up suicidal wishes is a way of controlling the therapist and receiving transference gratifications that are otherwise denied (Schwartz 1979; K. Smith: "Treating Suicidal Impulses Within a Psychotherapy," unpublished manuscript, 1993).

By nature most psychotherapists tend to feel an exaggerated responsibility for the welfare of their patients. The day-in and day-out suicidality of borderline patients may drive therapists to distraction. Their anxiety about whether or not the patient may act can compromise their ability to think clearly and reflectively about the meaning of the suicidality. The therapist's own sense of analytic space may get lost in the flurry of concern about what action should be taken to prevent the suicide. This collapse parallels the patient's failure to distinguish between impulsive actions and fantasy (Lewin and Schulz 1992). One of the therapist's ongoing tasks in the psychotherapeutic work with suicidal borderline patients is to assist the patient in constructing a symbolic dimension where fantasy and action are not the same thing. Therapists must help such patients see that their wish to die has specific meanings that can be understood through the psychotherapeutic process.

Obviously, in certain circumstances where the lethality of the patient is clear, therapists will have to take actions such as hospitalization to save the patient's life. But even in the context of providing structure to keep the patient alive, therapists must retain a psychological perspective on the meaning of what is transpiring. A distinction can be made between management of suicidality—involving the provision of protective structure or observation—and *treatment* of suicidality involving aggressive pharmacotherapy and a psychotherapeutic search for the underlying determinants of the wish to die (Gabbard 1994).

Lewin and Schulz (1992) pointed out that suicidality is not the same thing as suicide. Constant ruminations about the possibility of killing oneself may perform valuable psychological functions for the patient: "Suicidality, in fact, may be central to a patient's search for a degree of dignity and autonomy as well as connectedness worth staying alive to enjoy" (p. 237). If the therapist cannot make this empathic bridge to the patient's subjective use of suicidality as a mode of adaptation, the therapist may resort to a countertransference posture of decreased investment in the treatment and distance between himself or herself and the patient.

Another risk entailed by the therapist who fails to understand the value for the patient of remaining suicidal is to place too much emphasis on the elimination of suicidal ideation. Patients may feel terribly misunderstood by a therapist who seems hell-bent on removing all trace of suicidality. One exasperated borderline patient said to her therapist, "Look, doctor, I've been suicidal all my life! It's not going to go away in the next 5 minutes!" Such zeal in the therapist is another example of the therapist's own needs being placed before the patient's. Moreover, with intensely suicidal patients, such *furor therapeuticus* may have more ominous implications. A broad consensus exists among clinicians who treat suicidal patients that those who assume an omnipotent posture of being able to save their patients magically from killing themselves may unwittingly make the patient more lethal (Gabbard 1994; Hendin 1982; Meissner 1986; Richman and Eyman 1990; Searles 1967/1979; Zee 1972). Patients who are seriously suicidal have in common a deep-seated wish to be taken care of by an all-giving and all-loving, idealized parent (Richman and Eyman 1990; Smith and Eyman 1988).

Zealous efforts to save patients from themselves may lead patients on to think that a therapist is really a parent who is always available and always self-sacrificing. This form of therapist behavior provides patients with false hopes that will ultimately be dashed and lead them to further contemplation of suicide. Moreover, it colludes with borderline patients' tendency to assign to others the responsibility for keeping them alive, an aspect of behavior that Hendin (1982) characterized as one of the most lethal features of suicidal patients. When therapists place themselves in bondage to the patient, they will soon find that their omnipotent wishes are thwarted and consciously or unconsciously begin to wish the patient would disappear. Searles (1967) made the following observation:

> In the suicidal patient, who finds us so unable to be aware of the murderous feelings he fosters in us through his guilt- and anxiety-producing threats of suicide, feels increasingly constricted, perhaps indeed to the point of suicide, by the therapist who, in reaction formation against his intensifying, unconscious wishes to kill the patient, hovers increasingly "protectively" about the latter, for whom he feels an omnipotence-based physicianly concern. Hence it is, paradoxically, the very physician most anxiously concerned *to keep the patient alive* who tends most vigorously, at an unconscious level, to drive him to what has come to seem the only autonomous act left to him—namely, suicide. (p. 74)

There is little doubt that intensive psychotherapy of suicidal patients stirs sadistic and murderous wishes in the therapist. Chessick (1977) noted that the wish to kill the patient is usually the flip side of the fervent wish to rescue the patient. Therapists may fear that a patient's suicide will make them look bad to their colleagues, and they may feel resentful of the patient's power over them. It may not occur to the therapist that suicidal patients may attach to others only through sadomasochistic object ties (Maltsberger and Buie 1974).

From the foregoing comments, it should be obvious that the management of countertransference in the treatment of suicidal borderline patients is largely the management of countertransference hate. This may take the form of aversion or malice or a combination of both (Maltsberger and Buie 1974). The former may lead therapists to abandon the patient in subtle ways, such as forgetting appointments, forgetting to write orders for 15-minute rounds in hospital treatment, or withdrawing emotionally from the patient. Malicious impulses, on the other hand, may lead the therapist to be overtly hostile or sarcastic with the patient. Borderline patients realize that the therapist's narcissism is on the line when a patient is contemplating suicide. They may exploit this vulnerability by enjoying the sadistic power they wield over the therapist.

One principle of managing hate in the countertransference is prevention. By refusing to take the role of savior or omnipotent rescuer who will go to all forms of self-sacrifice to save the patient, therapists can avoid the resentment and hatred that goes along with that role. The second principle of managing countertransference hate with suicidal patients involves monitoring the defensive postures that one is likely to develop to deal with such hateful feelings. Maltsberger and Buie (1974) outlined five common defensive postures. First, one may repress the hate because it creates cognitive dissonance with the consciously valued role of a caring psychotherapist and have a conscious experience of being bored, restless, or inattentive. Second, the hatred may be turned against the self in the form of self-doubts and self-criticism for not doing a better job with the patient. Third, through reaction formation, the therapist may turn countertransference hate into its opposite and be oversolicitous in attempting to take care of the patient and tolerate extraordinary mistreatment by the patient. A fourth defensive posture is to project the countertransference hate into the patient and validate it by the many examples of negative transference brought to the treatment by the patient. The fifth defensive posture involves distorting or denying the validation of countertransference hate through devaluation of the patient or transferring the patient to another treater.

At some point in the long-term psychotherapy of a borderline patient, therapists commonly experience a profound sense of being trapped. The therapist may feel all alone in dealing with a serious suicide risk because the patient has exhausted all the resources in the community and can no longer pay for treatment. Local hospital units may deny admission to borderline patients who have refused to cooperate with treatment plans. Community mental health centers may feel burned out by such patients, and family members may have kicked the patient out of the house. At some level the therapist's feeling of being trapped is simply a reaction to the reality of external circumstances with the patient. At another level therapists may be experiencing an empathic identification with an aspect of the patient, who also feels trapped. Therapists must do their best to head off such developments by taking measures in advance to ensure that they do not end up as the only resource the patient has in the entire community. In addition, it is useful at the beginning of treatment to help the patient understand that psychotherapy alone may not be sufficient for the effective treatment and that other modalities and agencies must be available to mount an effective treatment strategy. In so doing, the therapist establishes the limits of psychotherapy from the outset.

The ultimate message in the psychotherapy of borderline patients is one of limits. When limits are communicated in an empathic and caring manner, a mourning process is facilitated. The treatment for hopelessness is not to instill false hope but to help the patient come to terms with authentic hopes related to what is realistically available from others. Another message that is implicit in acknowledging limits is that patients have some capacity to help themselves, especially in collaboration with an effective therapist. Tolerating frustration builds ego in borderline patients and will ultimately help them to overcome the sense of time urgency and delay impulse discharge. The mourning process also facilitates more balance between the paranoid-schizoid mode of functioning and the depressive mode, in which a balanced view of objects is more possible. The shift toward depressive functioning also facilitates the opening of analytic space so the patient can think symbolically about the meaning of the wish to be rescued.

Therapists must also reconcile themselves to the notion that certain patients may not be interested in giving up lifelong modes of adaptation such as chronic suicidality or sadomasochistic relatedness. A therapist's wish to change the patient may be perceived as the ultimate threat. Patients commonly dig in their heels and become more oppositional in the face of this external danger (Gabbard 1989). A helpful strategy in preventing disastrous countertransference enactments is to view the therapist's principal goal as to understand rather than to change. Two thousand years ago Seneca the Younger noted, "It is part of the cure to wish to be cured." It is not too late to heed his advice.

Summary

Physical, sexual, or verbal abuse and gross neglect are often involved in the etiology of borderline personality disorder. Specific countertransference patterns derive from the therapist's perception of the patient as a victim. These patterns can be viewed as a series of transference-countertransference enactments involving four principal characters in a psychotherapeutic drama: a victim, an abuser, an idealized and omnipotent rescuer, and an uninvolved mother. Through a projective-introjective process, these characters emerge in a series of complementary pairings between patient and therapist. Each of the characters represents an internal self- or object-representation within the patient, but the therapist's psychological predisposition to be a rescuer is also an important contributor to these enactments. Particularly when the patient is suicidal, therapists may become overzealous in their efforts to keep the patient alive and set themselves up to be tormented by gratifying the patient's demands. A fundamental component of managing countertransference is to help the patient deal with the therapist's limits.

References

Adler G: Borderline Psychopathology and Its Treatment. New York, Jason Aronson, 1985

Baker L, Silk KR, Westen D, et al: Malevolence, splitting, and parental ratings by borderlines. J Nerv Ment Dis 180:258–264, 1992

Bigras J, Biggs KH: Psychoanalysis as incestuous repetition: some technical considerations, in Adult Analysis and Childhood Sexual Abuse. Edited by Levine HB. Hillsdale, NJ, Analytic Press, 1990, pp 173–196

Bollas C: Forces of Destiny: Psychoanalysis and Human Idiom. Northvale, NJ, Jason Aronson, 1989

Chessick RD: Intensive Psychotherapy of the Borderline Patient. New York, Jason Aronson, 1977

Davies JM, Frawley MG: Dissociative processes and transference-countertransference paradigms in the psychoanalytically oriented treatment of adult survivors of childhood sexual abuse. Psychoanalytic Dialogues 2:5–36, 1992

Dupont J (ed): The Clinical Diary of Sandor Ferenczi. Translated by Ballint M, Jackson NZ. Cambridge, MA, Harvard University Press, 1988

Frank H, Paris J: Recollections of family experience in borderline patients. Arch Gen Psychiatry 38:1031–1034, 1981

Gabbard GO: The treatment of the "special patient" in a psychoanalytic hospital. International Review of Psychoanalysis 13:333–347, 1986

Gabbard GO: Patients who hate. Psychiatry 52:96–106, 1989

Gabbard GO: Commentary on "Dissociative Processes and Transference-Countertransference Paradigms . . . " by Jody Messler Davies and Mary Gail Frawley. Psychoanalytic Dialogues 2:37–47, 1992

Gabbard GO: Psychodynamic Psychiatry in Clinical Practice: The DSM-IV Edition. Washington, DC, American Psychiatric Press, 1994

Gabbard GO: When the patient is a therapist: special challenges in the analysis of mental health professionals. Psychoanal Rev (in press)

Goldberg RL, Mann LS, Wise TN, et al: Parental qualities as perceived by borderline personality disorders. Hillside J Clin Psychiatry 7:134–140, 1985

Grubrich-Simitis I: Six letters of Sigmund Freud and Sandor Ferenczi on the interrelationship of psychoanalytic theory and technique. International Review of Psychoanalysis 12:259–277, 1986

Hendin H: Psychotherapy and suicide, in Suicide in America. New York, WW Norton, 1982, pp 160–174

Herman JL, Perry JC, van der Kolk BA: Childhood trauma in borderline personality disorder. Am J Psychiatry 146:490–495, 1989

Hoffer A: The Freud-Ferenczi controversy—a living legacy. International Review of Psychoanalysis 18:465–472, 1991

Kernberg OF: Borderline Conditions and Pathological Narcissism. New York, Jason Aronson, 1975

Kluft R: Treating the patient who has been sexually exploited by a previous therapist. Psychiatr Clin North Am 12:483–500, 1989

Levine HB: Clinical issues in the analysis of adults who were sexually abused as children, in Adult Analysis and Childhood Sexual Abuse. Edited by Levine HB. Hillsdale, NJ, Analytic Press, 1990, pp 197–218

Lewin RA, Schulz CG: Losing and Fusing: Borderline and Transitional Object and Self Relations. Northvale, NJ, Jason Aronson, 1992

Lisman-Pieczanski N: Countertransference in the analysis of an adult who was sexually abused as a child, in Adult Analysis and Childhood Sexual Abuse. Edited by Levine HB. Hillsdale, NJ, Analytic Press, 1990, pp 137–147

Maltsberger JT, Buie DH: Countertransference hate in the treatment of suicidal patients. Arch Gen Psychiatry 30:625–633, 1974

Masterson JF, Rinsley DB: The borderline syndrome: the role of the mother in the genesis and psychic structure of the borderline personality. Int J Psychoanal 56:163–177, 1975

Meissner WW: Psychotherapy and the Paranoid Process. Northvale, NJ, Jason Aronson, 1986

Nigg JT, Silk KR, Westen D, et al: Object representations in the early memories of sexually abused borderline patients. Am J Psychiatry 148:864–869, 1991

Ogata SN, Silk KR, Goodrich S, et al: Childhood sexual and physical abuse in adult patients with borderline personality disorder. Am J Psychiatry 147:1008–1013, 1990

Ogden TH: The Primitive Edge of Experience. Northvale, NJ, Jason Aronson, 1989

Paris J, Frank H: Perceptions of parental bonding in borderline patients. Am J Psychiatry 146:1498–1499, 1989

Richman J, Eyman JR: Psychotherapy of suicide: individual, group, and family approaches, in Understanding Suicide: The State of the Art. Edited by Lester D. Philadelphia, PA, Charles C Thomas, 1990, pp 139–158

Schwartz DA: The suicidal character. Psychiatr Q 51:64–70, 1979

Searles HF: The "dedicated physician" in the field of psychotherapy and psychoanalysis (1967), in Countertransference and Related Subjects. Madison, CT, International Universities Press, 1979, pp 71–88

Smith K, Eyman J: Ego structure and object differentiation in suicidal patients, in Primitive Mental States of the Rorschach. Edited by Lerner HD, Lerner PM. Madison, CT, International Universities Press, 1988, pp 175–202

Soloff PH, Millward JW: Developmental histories of borderline patients. Compr Psychiatry 24:574–588, 1983

Stone MH: The Fate of Borderline Patients: Successful Outcome and Psychiatric Practice. New York, Guilford, 1990

Sussman MB: A Curious Calling: Unconscious Motivations for Practicing Psychotherapy. Northvale, NJ, Jason Aronson, 1992

Walsh F: Family study 1976: 14 new borderline cases, in Chapter 5—The family of the borderline patient, in The Borderline Patient. Edited by Grinker RR, Werble B. New York, Jason Aronson, 1977

Westen D, Ludolph P, Misle B, et al: Physical and sexual abuse in adolescent girls with borderline personality disorder. Am J Orthopsychiatry 60:55–66, 1990

Zanarini MC, Gunderson JG, Marino MF, et al: Childhood experiences of borderline patients. Compr Psychiatry 30:18–25, 1989

Zee HJ: Blindspots in recognizing serious suicidal intentions. Bull Menninger Clin 36:551–555, 1972

Zweig-Frank H, Paris J: Parents' emotional neglect and overprotection according to the recollections of patients with borderline personality disorder. Am J Psychiatry 148:648–651, 1991

CHAPTER 4

On Holding, Containment, and Thinking One's Own Thoughts

B ecause of the centrality of projective identification in the experience of treating borderline patients, therapists often feel invaded and transformed into someone other than who they are. Attempting to resist this transformative process can be a formidable problem. As Masterson (1976) noted, "Probably the single most difficult skill to acquire in psychotherapy of borderline patients is the ability to recognize and control one's own identification with their projections" (p. 342).

The following clinical vignette illustrates how the projected aspects of the patient can "sneak up" on therapists and seem to take over before they know what has happened.

[Ms. W telling Mr. D, a clinical social worker, that she would not go back to the hospital unit at the end of the session.]

Ms. W: There's nothing for me on the unit. Nobody likes me there. Nobody has ever liked me. What's wrong with me, Mr. D? Why has no one ever liked me? It seems so hopeless. It's never going to change. Why should I go on?

Mr. D: Right now you feel hopeless. You sound like you're on the verge of despair. You need to be in a protected environment.

Ms. W: How is that going to help me? I've been this way for 10 years. How will being in the hospital unit over the weekend help me? Nothing's going to change.

71

Mr. D: For one thing, it may help you avoid harming yourself.

Ms. W: I don't think I need to be in a hospital.

Mr. D: Do you feel like killing yourself now?

Ms. W [angrily]: Why are you asking me that? What a stupid question! I've felt like killing myself for 10 years. There's never a day when I don't feel like killing myself.

Mr. D felt an inexplicable sense of rage coming over him. He felt the patient was an ungrateful wretch. He was merely trying to protect her from suicide, and she was treating him with utter contempt. His sense that the patient was biting the hand that was attempting to feed her made him respond in an impulsive and hostile manner.

Mr. D: Why are you getting so nasty with me now? You know I only asked because I'm concerned about your safety.

Ms. W [crying]: Now *you* think I'm nasty! See? No one likes me. Even you think I'm bad. Why shouldn't I kill myself? Nobody likes me. What's wrong with me?

Mr. D was suddenly filled with remorse when he saw how his comment had devastated Ms. W. He felt he had made a terrible gaff, and he wondered what had gotten into him. He felt he was acting in a way that was "not like himself." He rapidly moved to make amends to the patient.

Mr. D: I probably shouldn't have used the word *nasty.* What I was reacting to is how angry you got at me for expressing concern about your hurting yourself.

Ms. W: No, it's true. I am nasty. That's why everybody hates me. You feel the same way everybody else does toward me. I might as well die. It's so painful to go on living.

Mr. D: I still would like to know if you have any plans to kill yourself. I know it makes you angry for me to ask, but I am concerned, and I need to know how you're feeling.

Ms. W [after a pause]: I probably won't.

Mr. D: What do you mean, "probably"?

Ms. W: I don't think I'll be able to buy a gun over the weekend, and that's the only way I'd do it.

Mr. D once again felt a sense of rage welling up within him. He felt he was being toyed with. But this time he sat with the feeling rather than impulsively lashing out at the patient. He entered into an internal monologue that went something like this:

> She is being an incredible pain in the ass. For some reason she's trying to provoke me into attacking her again and telling her how obnoxious she is. Why does she want me to be hateful like everyone else? I'm attempting to be different and look out for her welfare, and she insists on making me into a monster like her husband. I'd like to tell her off, but I need to bite my tongue. What's developing here between us is incredibly important for the treatment, if I can just keep from acting on it.

Ms. W: If I go back to the hospital unit, I want one thing in return from you. Would you please talk to Dr. V about giving me permission to drive my car?

Mr. D felt a sense of calm and composure coming over him and was able to reflect dispassionately on the manipulation attempt by Ms. W.

Mr. D: I'm not in any position to make bargains. You'll need to discuss that with Dr. V. I do think, though, that as long as you're wanting to buy a gun, it's important that you're in a protected environment. Now, let's go back to the unit together.

On Thinking One's Own Thoughts

In this exchange between Ms. W and Mr. D, a familiar pattern in the psychotherapy of borderline patients emerges. Mr. D feels so controlled by the patient's projective identification that he is no longer thinking his own thoughts nor feeling "like himself." Lewin and Schulz (1992) analogized this phenomenon to ventriloquism: "Often it is the therapist who is the ventriloquist's dummy, speaking lines that have been written by a borderline patient who remains aloof and untouched, quite unaware that he is the impresario of the performance" (p. 37).

Projective identification is a powerful form of direct communication that collapses the analytic space (Ogden 1986; Winnicott

1971). This highly coercive force operates primarily within the paranoid-schizoid mode of mental functioning and therefore disables the therapist's ability to reflect on meanings and assign them to one's subjective state. Therapists in the throes of projective identification find that they are locked into a "dance" with the patient that is inevitable and obligatory. In this situation they cannot think their own thoughts because they have been transformed into a repudiated part of the patient. Mr. D felt he could not prevent himself from calling the patient "nasty" and reacting with a sense of hurt and outrage at the patient's treatment of him. He felt that some form of action was necessary to unload the powerful feelings he was experiencing, and the action came in the form of a sarcastic comment to Ms. W.

Symington (1990) described communication of this sort as a process in which one person "bullies" another, who feels like a victim of the bully. He made a distinction between *reacting* and *responding*. Reacting is a knee-jerk, instinctual mode of communication, in which one is unable to think one's own thoughts because of being forced into thinking someone else's thoughts. Symington, elaborating on Bion's (1984) thinking, made the point that a central goal of the therapist's activity is to achieve freedom in the realm of thought: "A person who is able to think his own thoughts is free. When someone cannot think his own thoughts he is not free" (p. 96). Within this context he stressed that therapists must resist the pressure to react and must tolerate the coercive power of intense affects until they shift into a responding mode. Just as a mother transforms the primitive anxieties of her baby through the process of her own reverie, therapists must metabolize the affects of the patient sufficiently so that they can think their own thoughts and speak to the patient from a cognitive and affective center within themselves rather than from a projected part of the patient.

Another aspect of the exchange between Ms. W and Mr. D that is typical of psychotherapy with borderline patients is that a therapist may have to react before responding. Mr. D learned something from the first instance of provocation so that when he began to feel provoked the second time, he was able to "hold" the feeling rather than react with knee-jerk impulsiveness. One of the crucial elements in the management of countertransference is to achieve a state of freedom in which therapists can think their own thoughts. However, this ambitious goal involves an ongoing process of "working back" to one's own center of being from a position of having been taken over by the patient and thinking aspects of the patient's thoughts. This process is variously referred to as holding and containing in the literature, and this chapter is devoted to a systematic analysis of the therapist's activities that constitute the process.

On Holding and Containment

To a large extent the successful (and therapeutic) management of countertransference in the treatment of borderline patients depends on two functions—holding and containment. *Holding* is a term that derives from Winnicott's (1965) notion that a mother provides a specific form of environment that facilitates an infant's growth. Through interactions between a mother and her infant, a shared transitional space is created in which the infant ultimately internalizes holding functions performed by the mother. The term *containment* stems from Bion's (1984) description of how the mother processes the affects of her infant. The mother bears the uncontainable affects of her baby, and through her reverie, she detoxifies and transforms the affects into a form that allows the infant to reintroject and tolerate them. In Ogden's (1982) formulation of projective identification discussed in Chapter 1, the "psychological processing" in the third step approximates what Bion referred to as containment.

Although holding and containing are distinct and arise from disparate theoretical sources, the therapist's functions that are associated with the two terms have considerable overlap. Some authors (D. E. Scharff 1992; Scharff and Scharff 1992) have stressed that holding was used by Winnicott (1965) to refer to an interpersonal phenomenon occurring in the external world, in contrast to Bion's (1984) use of containment, which described an intrapsychic process in the mother. Other authors, such as Casement (1985), use the terms synonymously: "In more human terms, what is needed is a form of holding, such as a mother gives to her distressed child. There are various ways in which one adult can offer to another this holding (or containment)" (p. 133). Both terms imply an alternative to action—a postponement of impulsive reaction to the patient in the service of bearing and processing powerful feelings generated in the patient-therapist dyad. The twin processes of holding and containment transform therapists in such a way that they can *respond* rather than *react,* and think their own thoughts rather than someone else's.

The term *holding* has been problematic in contemporary usage because of its being interpreted literally in some quarters. Holding certainly evokes an image of a screaming baby being embraced and soothed by a calm and comforting mother. Indeed, some accounts of Winnicott's actual behavior in treatment situations indicate that he physically held a patient's hand over an extended time (Little 1990). However, the very essence of the notion of holding is a movement from the concrete to the symbolic. This concept provides a supportive context in which patients who are entertaining concrete actions and impulses can translate them into fantasies and ideas to be "played with" and reflected on rather than discarded. In the mother-infant model of Winnicott (1965), the mother performs functions of which the infant is incapable. The holding environment provides a form of modeling for the infant (or patient) so that capacities of the mother (or therapist) can be observed and ultimately internalized. Lewin and Schulz (1992) stressed that a holding environment cannot actually hold the patient unless the patient allows it to, and in that sense, holding should be viewed as a joint construction project from both the therapist's side and the patient's side. They link holding to projective identification as well, and they conceptualize the therapist as taking unbearable aspects of the patient into a kind of safe deposit box until the patient is more adequately equipped for the return of the emotionally charged contents.

The images evoked by the concept of holding also have led some to misconstrue the term as endorsing an unconditionally loving, soothing, and caring attitude in the therapist. Although Winnicott (1954–1955, 1963) stressed that the mother must meet the infant's needs, he also emphasized that the mothering must not be too good. Only through frustration and disillusionment can the infant ultimately grow. From the standpoint of the therapist-patient dyad, patients must be able to experience their therapists as imperfect objects so that they can reexperience the externalization of old internal object relationships. How can a patient work through problems that occur in the context of real human relationships in the presence of a saintly and endlessly patient therapist?

This clarification of the meaning of holding also implies that therapists must set limits in certain situations. As reflected in the discussion of negotiating a contractual understanding with the patient in Chapter 2, therapists must not create an expectation of limitless supplies. Nor should they allow themselves to be the masochistic victims of sadistic and unrelenting abuse from the patient. A holding environment is one in which the rights of others are respected.

Holding also involves surviving. Winnicott (1968) believed that the therapist's survival of the borderline patient's destructive attacks is a crucial element in helping the patient to make use of the therapist as a truly external object outside the patient's omnipotent control. He drew a developmental analogy in this regard by noting that the mother must survive the primitive attacks of the infant for the child to proceed with development and maturation. Holding, then, also involves surviving over time while the patient renounces internal objects and comes to see the therapist as a real external object separate from the patient's internal world (Ogden 1986).

In Bion's (1959) original use of containment, he was addressing the need for the mother to help the infant avoid unmanageable pain. He felt if the mother did not serve as a container of the infant's anxieties, she would be in the position of dumping unmodified forms of anxiety back into the infant before the infant was ready to handle them. Outside the therapeutic context, borderline patients frequently experience an analogous process in which the affects they arouse in others are neither contained nor modified but simply forced back down the patient's throat. In the therapist-patient dyad, this may happen in the form of interpretation or avoidance.

Bion (1959) believed that when the mother returns unmodified affects to the infant, the infant is likely to feel persecuted by the return of the projected contents and may experience a fragmentation of the self as a result. Similarly, borderline patients often feel persecuted by therapists who are unable to contain, as illustrated by Ms. W's reaction to Mr. D's exhortation that she was being "nasty." When therapists are capable of containing the patient's unbearable feelings, patients will ultimately learn that the nameless dread is not as horrible as what they might have imagined. Watching the therapist struggle with the same affects as the patient ultimately diffuses that dread (Casement 1985).

Although containment is often presented as an alternative to interpretation or a way of postponing interpretation (Gabbard 1991; Winnicott 1968), the two generally work in tandem in the psychotherapy process. A period of containment may be necessary before the therapist can effectively and empathically interpret what is going in the patient. Viewing containment as inferior to interpretation would certainly be erroneous in terms of its therapeutic potential. Since borderline patients are often stuck in a paranoid-schizoid psychological mode, projective identification is their main mode of communication. The only way the therapist can "hang in there" is to contain what is being communicated and hold it until the patient can more readily reintroject the projected contents and understand an interpretive formulation.

Containment should not be equated with a kind of passive inaction (Rosenfeld 1987). Nor should it be understood as masochistically enduring the patient's attacks (Ogden 1982). Containment involves silent processing, but it also entails verbal clarifications of what is going on inside the patient and what is transpiring in the patient-therapist dyad. Although containment is often applied to situations in which the therapist's negatively charged affects are mobilized, it applies equally to the technical handling of more positively tinged affects and introjects, as illustrated by the following case example:

> Ms. V was seeing Dr. E during her regular therapist's summer vacation. She was growing increasingly attached to Dr. E, while becoming more and more disenchanted with her regular therapist.

Ms. V: I just don't know if I can go back to Dr. U [her regular therapist] after these last 2 weeks with you. It reminds me of the old song, "How Are You Going to Keep Them Down on the Farm After They've Seen Paree." You have the qualities I need in a therapist. You're kind and compassionate. I feel you really listen to me. You're not nearly as narcissistic as Dr. U. You also have about 10 more years of experience than he does, and I think you'd agree that I need an experienced therapist.

As Dr. E listened to the flattering words of Ms. V, he found himself struggling with a conflicting set of feelings. She seemed so genuine and poignant in the way she spoke and in the way she looked at him. His internal monologue went something like this:

She's probably right. Dr. U is a kind of stuffy, self-absorbed guy who has difficulty conveying to others that he's really listening. I *am* much more experienced than he is and probably a better therapist overall. Is this an idealizing transference or simply a smart patient who is able to make discriminating judgments about people? There's something about her that is enormously appealing. I have the feeling that I could really help her if given the chance. Maybe I should talk to Dr. U about the possibility of transferring her to me, if that's what she really wants. On the other hand, I'm probably allowing myself to be seduced. This kind of splitting and idealization occurs all the time when one therapist is covering for another. I'm sure I'd fall off the pedestal in due time. And yet, there seems to be something incredibly special about the kind of communication we've established in only 2 weeks. What am I doing? I feel like I'm falling under her spell.

Ms. V: I know someone else who was in treatment with you, and she said you were the best thing that ever happened to her. She said that if I could talk you into taking me as a patient, it would be an incredibly smart thing to do. I think that there's a kind of "chemistry" factor in finding the right therapist. I don't have it with Dr. U, but I clearly do have it with you. It's just like with certain men I have an instant attraction, whereas others do nothing for me even though they are caring and decent guys.

As Dr. E continued to listen silently, he reflected on his own contribution to the countertransference longings he was experiencing. He instantly flashed on a woman in his past he had once dated. Ms. V bore a striking resemblance to that woman and re-created in him a sense that he was being sucked back into that ill-fated relationship. Just as he had wanted to rescue the woman from his past, he now was wanting to rescue Ms. V. He also noted the strong sense of competitiveness with Dr. U, who he wanted to show up by being a better therapist to Ms. V. The more he analyzed the "spell" he was under, the more he mastered the situation and began to think his own thoughts instead of those engendered by Ms. V.

In the foregoing vignette, we can see how the containment process really involves a host of interrelated internal processes. In describing Bion's conception of containment, Grotstein (1981) compared it to the activity of a prism:

> Bion's conception is of an elaborated primary process activity which acts like a *prism* to refract the intense hue of the infant's screams into the components of the color spectrum, so to speak, so as to sort them out and relegate them to a hierarchy of importance and of mental action. Thus, containment for Bion is a very active process which involves feeling, thinking, organizing, and acting. Silence would be the least part of it. (p. 134)

The activities of a therapist who is involved in containing can be subdivided into several interrelated functions.

Diagnosis of the Patient's Internal Object Relations

In the midst of the chaos and ambiguity generated by the patient-therapist interaction, the therapist will gradually become aware of specific aspects of the patient's internal world. In intensive psychotherapy of borderline patients, countertransference is often the most reliable approach to diagnostic understanding (Searles 1986). For example, Dr. E's growing awareness of the transference-countertransference situation between him and Ms. V helped him recognize an enactment of a specific object relationship involving an idealized rescuing object and a helpless, seductive self in need of rescue. In the case of Ms. W and Mr. D, a sadomasochistic internal object relationship was diagnosed through the therapist's ability to learn from his impulsive response to Ms. W's provocation.

The recognition of these transference-countertransference enactments considerably precedes the patient's ability to understand them and use interpretations of them in a constructive manner. Therefore, therapists must postpone the need to interpret while systematically scrutinizing their countertransference long before the patient can put words to feelings. Bion (1974) made the following observation:

> Psycho-analysts must be able to tolerate the differences or the difficulties of the analysand long enough to recognise what they are. If psycho-analysts are to be able to interpret what the analysand says, they must have a great capacity for tolerating their analysands' statements without rushing to the conclusion that they know the interpretations. (p. 72)

Internal Supervision

In Dr. E's inner narrative, a "supervisor" was clearly at work. The therapist was recognizing a countertransference problem, commenting on a splitting process involving devaluation of the previous therapist and idealization of the substitute, and helping himself think more clearly about what was going on. Casement (1985) referred to this process as *internal supervision*. He noted that it originates when therapists are immersed in their own treatment experience and find "that island of contemplation—from which they could observe with their analyst what they were experiencing in the transference" (p. 31). All therapists need the experience of being a patient to learn, among other things, the process of observing oneself. Casement suggested that trial identifications with the patient through empathy are an important part of this internal supervision function and of containment as well. Therapists empathically place themselves in the shoes of the patient and "try on" aspects of the patient's internal world to understand more effectively what is happening in the transference situation.

Achievement of an Analytic Space

Intimately related to Casement's (1985) concept of internal supervision is achieving a state of double consciousness. When therapists undergo their own treatment, what they learn as patients is the experience of the transference as both real and illusory. One part of them participates in a reenactment of a past object relationship; another part observes the reenactment and reflects on it. Sterba (1934) referred to this fundamental state of consciousness as *ego dissociation*. In a more contemporary context, Ogden (1986) referred to this state of double consciousness as *analytic space*. As noted earlier, the patient's projective identification tends to collapse the therapist's analytic space just as it does the patient's. Therapists must first reopen their own capacity to participate in an enactment while reflecting on it before the patient can be helped to do the same. The optimal state of mind for therapists is when they can allow themselves to be "sucked in" to the patient's world while retaining the ability to observe it happening in front of their eyes. In such a state, therapists are truly thinking their own thoughts, even though they are under the patient's influence to some extent.

Self-Analysis

Therapists are containing not only the patient's affects but also their own countertransference responses. Therefore, systematic self-analysis must be a part of an effective containment effort. Specifically, therapists must examine their own contributions to the intense feelings generated in the dyad. As we noted in Chapter 1, projective identification involves an introjective process by the therapist that, to some extent, is based on whether or not the projected contents of the patient are "a good fit" with the therapist's own internal self- and object-representations (J. S. Scharff 1992). Therapists who, like Dr. E, feel "under the spell" of the patient need to reflect on how the evoked response generated by the patient interfaces with their own intrapsychic needs. Dr. E was able to identify in himself a powerful need to rescue that perfectly complemented Ms. V's need to be rescued. Moreover, through following his own associations in a self-analytic process, he could identify a similarity between Ms. V and an important female relationship from his past. This self-analytic process typically goes on between sessions as well as during sessions as the therapist analyzes dreams, daydreams, and other thoughts that occur about the patient in the course of the work week.

Silent Interpretation

This discussion of holding and containment should make clear that neither interpretation nor containment alone is sufficient for the psychotherapy of borderline patients. Both must work together to help the patient gain sufficient understanding and experience to effect change. However, timing is of the utmost importance in interpretation. When interpretation is used to unload affects or other projected contents from the therapist to the patient, the patient may experience it as an attack and be unable to listen to the meaning of the interpretation. Hence, one valuable aspect of containment is silent interpretation (Gabbard 1989). Similar to how therapists diagnose the patient's internal object relations based on the processing of the projective identifications going on, they can also formulate their understanding of the patient's difficulties and the dynamic-genetic explanations that are relevant while they contain. These interpretations are formulated as part of the internal narrative and supervision process going on within the therapist's mind and are verbalized when the patient is in a receptive analytic space so that the explanation and understanding provided can be reflected on and assimilated.

Verbal Clarification

Too much silence can create considerable difficulties in the psycho-therapy of borderline patients. Many are prone to experience the therapist's silence as abandonment or lack of concern. Some bor-derline patients will become increasingly paranoid as they project the worst possible meanings into the therapist's silence. For this reason it is important that the containment process not be carried out in total silence. Verbal clarifications of what is going on and invitations to expand on feelings and perceptions the patient is ex-periencing are essential to keep the process from deteriorating. For example, in the vignette involving Ms. V, Dr. E might have said, "Can you tell me more about how you perceive me as so different from Dr. U?" A typical clarification might be, "So it sounds like you're saying that working with me for 2 weeks has made you aware of differences in the styles of Dr. U and me." This kind of statement or question does not challenge the patient's view but merely invites further elaboration.

Beyond Psychotherapy

Most of our discussion of holding and containment has been geared to the psychotherapeutic situation. However, only a minority of borderline patients will be able to derive a sufficient degree of holding from psychotherapy alone. The majority will require a much expanded version of the holding environment. Indeed, the viability of a psychotherapy process may depend on the nature and extent of adjunctive holding environments from which the patient can seek support between psychotherapy sessions. The borderline patient's impaired capacity for self-regulation (Grotstein 1987) may create pressures for others besides psychotherapists to serve as con-tainers and regulators of the patient's affective states.

At one extreme we find patients with extraordinarily severe and unremitting problems who can only be treated in the context of extended hospital treatment (Gabbard 1992a, 1994). In this sub-group, patients are unremittingly suicidal and/or self-destructive and may require a more literal form of holding, such as physical restraints to prevent self-injury and 24-hour special observation status. Others in this group create such overwhelming countertransference problems in treaters that individual psychotherapy as an outpatient is not tenable. Marcus (1987) described this indication for extended hospital treatment as follows:

> The problem with the sickest patients is that the affects are uncontainable by a single individual. The affects are more easily containable by the group, because at any one moment some members are not under direct threat and therefore can maintain observing ego. (p. 251)

Such patients will re-create their internal object world in the milieu of the inpatient unit through projective identification (Gabbard 1986, 1988, 1989, 1992b, 1994). In this form of intensive psychoanalytically oriented hospital treatment, the inpatient staff collectively contain the projected aspects of the patient and must work together as a cohesive group to process and detoxify those contents before returning them to the patient. The structure of the inpatient program, the limits that are set by the nursing staff, and the concern of the entire therapeutic community are also components of the holding environment of a psychiatric hospital. In addition, some borderline patients may view medication as a somewhat concrete and psychologically external form of holding (Lewin and Schulz 1992).

Most borderline patients can get by with periodic brief hospitalizations to reorganize and then continue their outpatient psychotherapy. Others may need a day hospital program to extend the containment provided in psychotherapy. Many of the same holding functions of an inpatient unit are provided by a day hospital; however, to utilize such a setting, patients must be able to have a sufficient capacity for self-regulation and self-soothing so that they can live independently during evenings and nights. Support groups such as Alcoholics Anonymous, Narcotics Anonymous, and Overeaters Anonymous may also provide forms of holding for borderline patients.

Inherent in this discussion of extrapsychotherapeutic forms of holding is the notion that psychotherapists themselves may need an external holding environment to manage intense countertransference states stirred up by unbearable affects in the patient. A treatment team in an inpatient unit or a day hospital, or even an improvised network of treaters in an outpatient setting, provides a holding environment for all the treaters. We all have countertransference blind spots that only others can see, so one function of a treatment team is to hold a mirror up to treaters and point out countertransference enactments that go unnoticed by individuals.

For this reason, solo practitioners with predominantly outpatient psychotherapy have developed peer support groups that meet once a month—sometimes over dinner or at breakfast—to discuss countertransference problems. As we discuss in some detail in Chapter 9, a supervisor or consultant can be a valuable resource to contain the therapist's feelings. The essential point to underscore in this context is that psychotherapists must never feel that they are all alone in the "lion's den" with a difficult patient. Professional isolation is a setup for the most dire forms of countertransference acting out that ruin careers and destroy lives.

Summary

Therapists who are locked in the throes of projective identification with a borderline patient often find that they cannot think their own thoughts because they have been transformed into a disavowed part of the patient. This obligatory sense of *reacting* must gradually be transformed to a *responding* mode. Through holding and containment, therapists can metabolize and "detoxify" the powerful affects evoked by the patient and work their way back to their own autonomous center of thinking and feeling. Holding and containment should not be construed as passive inaction, masochistic enduring of the patient's attacks, or active soothing. These concepts entail a series of interrelated functions, including diagnosis of the patient's internal object relations through studying one's own countertransference responses, internal supervision, self-analysis, silent interpretation, verbal clarification, and the achievement of a state of double consciousness, often referred to as *analytic space*. Therapists must allow themselves to be "sucked in" to the patient's world while still maintaining their observing capacity. The notion of creating a holding environment transcends the psychotherapeutic dyad and also applies to hospital or partial hospital treatment in which both patients and treaters may require a holding environment to create an effective milieu.

References

Bion WR: Attacks on linking (1959), in Second Thoughts: Selected Papers on Psycho-Analysis. New York, Jason Aronson, 1984, pp 93–109

Bion WR: Second Thoughts: Selected Papers on Psycho-Analysis. New York, Jason Aronson, 1984

Bion WR: Bion's Brazilian Lectures 1. Rio de Janeiro, Imago Editora, 1974

Casement P: On Learning From the Patient. London, Tavistock, 1985

Gabbard GO: The treatment of the "special" patient in a psychoanalytic hospital. International Review of Psychoanalysis 13:333–347, 1986

Gabbard GO: A contemporary perspective on psychoanalytically informed hospital treatment. Hosp Community Psychiatry 39:1291–1295, 1988

Gabbard GO: On "doing nothing" in the psychoanalytic treatment of the refractory borderline patient. Int J Psychoanal 70:527–534, 1989

Gabbard GO: Technical approaches to transference hate in the analysis of borderline patients. Int J Psychoanal 72:625–637, 1991

Gabbard GO: Comparative indications for brief and extended hospitalization, in American Psychiatric Press Review of Psychiatry, Vol 11. Edited by Tasman A, Riba MB. Washington, DC, American Psychiatric Press, 1992a, pp 503–517

Gabbard GO: The therapeutic relationship in psychiatric hospital treatment. Bull Menninger Clin 56:4–19, 1992b

Gabbard GO: Psychodynamic Psychiatry in Clinical Practice: The DSM-IV Edition. Washington, DC, American Psychiatric Press, 1994

Grotstein JS: Splitting and Projective Identification. New York, Jason Aronson, 1981

Grotstein JS: The borderline as a disorder of self-regulation, in The Borderline Patient: Emerging Concepts in Diagnosis, Psychodynamics, and Treatment, Vol 1. Edited by Grotstein JS, Solomon MF, Lang JA. Hillsdale, NJ, Analytic Press, 1987, pp 347–383

Lewin RA, Schulz CG: Losing and Fusing: Borderline and Transitional Object and Self Relations. Northvale, NJ, Jason Aronson, 1992

Little MI: Psychotic Anxieties and Containment: A Personal Record of an Analysis With Winnicott. Northvale, NJ, Jason Aronson, 1990

Marcus E: Relationship of illness and intensive hospital treatment to length of stay. Psychiatr Clin North Am 10:247–255, 1987

Masterson JF: Psychotherapy of the Borderline Adult: A Developmental Approach. New York, Brunner/Mazel, 1976

Ogden TH: Projective Identification and Psychotherapeutic Technique. New York, Jason Aronson, 1982

Ogden TH: The Matrix of the Mind: Object Relations and the Psychoanalytic Dialogue. Northvale, NJ, Jason Aronson, 1986

Rosenfeld H: Impasse and Interpretation: Therapeutic and Anti-Therapeutic Factors in the Psychoanalytic Treatment of Psychotic, Borderline, and Neurotic Patients. London, Tavistock, 1987

Scharff DE: Refinding the Object and Reclaiming the Self. Northvale, NJ, Jason Aronson, 1992

Scharff JS: Projective and Introjective Identification and the Use of the Therapist's Self. Northvale, NJ, Jason Aronson, 1992

Scharff JS, Scharff DE: Scharff Notes: A Primer of Object Relations Therapy. Northvale, NJ, Jason Aronson, 1992

Searles HF: My Work With Borderline Patients. Northvale, NJ, Jason Aronson, 1986

Sterba R: The fate of the ego in analytic therapy. Int J Psychoanal 15:117–126, 1934

Symington N: The possibility of human freedom and its transmission (with particular reference to the thought of Bion). Int J Psychoanal 71:95–106, 1990

Winnicott DW: The depressive position in normal development (1954–1955), in Collected Papers: Through Paediatrics to Psycho-Analysis. New York, Basic Books, 1958, pp 262–277

Winnicott DW: Communicating and not communicating leading to a study of certain opposites (1963), in The Maturational Process and the Facilitating Environment: Studies in the Theory of Emotional Development. New York, International Universities Press, 1965, pp 179–192

Winnicott DW: The Maturational Process and the Facilitating Environment: Studies in the Theory of Emotional Development. New York, International Universities Press, 1965

Winnicott DW: Playing and Reality. New York, Basic Books, 1971

Winnicott DW: The use of an object and relating through identification (1968), in Psycho-Analytic Exploration. Edited by Winnicott C, Shepherd R, Davis M. Cambridge, MA, Harvard University Press, 1989, pp 218–227

CHAPTER 5

Reactions to
Rage and Hatred

One of the most challenging features intrinsic to the psychotherapy of borderline patients is the necessity of withstand-
ing raw expressions of rage and hatred. Many therapists may be
drawn to the field, at least in part, because the practice of psychotherapy itself serves as a reaction formation against sadism, hatred,
and aggression (Gabbard 1991; McLaughlin 1961; Menninger
1957; Schafer 1954). Being the object of unrelenting hatred and
anger tends to erode our carefully constructed defenses against hating our patients. When a therapist's efforts to be helpful and to
provide understanding are greeted with contempt, the clinician
may feel that the whole psychotherapeutic endeavor is not worth
the toll it entails. The conscious altruistic wishes with which most
therapists enter the field are thwarted by a patient who is biting the
feeding hand.

A particularly disconcerting aspect of the transference aggression one experiences with borderline patients is that it may be triggered by the slightest provocation. The *pars pro toto* reaction
described in Chapter 1 stems from a form of splitting in which the
therapist is perceived as "all good" or "all bad" (Kernberg 1975). An
idealized therapist can fall from the pedestal in the twinkling of an
eye as a result of one slight misstep. The following vignette
illustrates a common scenario:

> *Ms. U:* I want Bill so badly. I think he was quiet and distant
> when he saw me at the bar with Mark [her long-time boy-

friend] because he really is attracted to me. I'm sure of it. The way he looks at me tells me that he wants me. I could have him if I wanted him. I know I could. He knows I'm jealous of Jane.

As Ms. U went on and on about how Bill was secretly attracted to her, Dr. F became rather bored and realized that he had not been listening to what she was saying. When he realized that his attention had become distracted, he blinked and refocused on the patient's words.

Ms. U [shouting]: I'm boring you! You really don't care!
Dr. F: You've suddenly shifted gears.
Ms. U: You blinked!

The patient delivered her observation in the form of an accusation, as if Dr. F's blinking was the most heinous of acts.

Ms. U [now more seriously and angrily]: This therapy isn't working! You don't care. This is obviously not a good match. You don't give me insights. You don't talk about my envy! I can't develop a relationship with you. It's no use to keep at this!

Dr. F groaned inwardly. The complaints he was hearing were part of a familiar litany about how he should change to meet the patient's needs. He felt completely controlled by the patient, so that he did not even have the freedom to blink or shift his attention away from Ms. U without being blasted for it.

Dr. F: A few minutes ago you wanted me to hold you. I haven't changed. Something inside of you has changed.
Ms. U: No it hasn't. I don't think this can work. You don't give me insights. You talk about my jealousy. I can't develop a relationship with you.
Dr. F: I think you were trying to connect with me by telling me about the men in your life, and you felt rejected when I blinked.
Ms. U: Yes, I did! You don't talk about my fears. You don't care about me!
Dr. F: You seem very sensitive to being rejected. Rather than considering the variety of reasons why I might blink, you assume I'm rejecting you.
Ms. U: You seem pretty together. You're well educated, you're at-

tractive, you dress well, and you're happily married, I'm sure. I have none of those things. I could have them if I didn't have such problems. I think you know what's wrong with me, but you're not telling me. How can I possibly manage better when I don't even know what's wrong?

Dr. F: For what reason would I withhold important information from you?

Ms. U: Oh, you're not withholding? Then you don't know, do you? That's even worse! Oh, my God, what's going to happen to me? You're only guessing! I'm lost. You're lost, too. We're both lost.

Ms. U's words felt like an indictment, or more accurately, a guilty verdict, regarding the therapist's inadequacies. Dr. F considered spewing forth a fancy diagnostic formulation to vindicate himself and supposedly satisfy the patient, but he chose not to, realizing that he was simply getting increasingly defensive in response to the accusations. Instead, he opted to highlight the inconsistencies in the patient's demands.

Dr. F: A moment ago I was pretty together.

Ms. U: [angry silence]

Dr. F: You put so much energy into arranging the external world and your relationships.

Ms. U: I have to! I'll fall apart if I don't do that.

Dr. F: That's a good reason. But you overlook what happens inside. I think there's a process of unconsciously externalizing what's going on inside and then seeing it in others. . . .

Dr. F stopped himself in mid-sentence when he realized that he was under the influence of a countertransference pull to give a highly intellectualized and abstract explanation for what was going on with his patient.

Dr. F: I'm sorry, I think I've gotten a bit abstract here.

Ms. U: Go on, I was following your explanation.

Dr. F [wondering how the patient could follow what was making no sense to him]: Really, I don't think it's helpful to continue with such intellectualized ideas.

Ms. U: You don't think that I'm capable of understanding, do you? Just because you have a fancy degree.

Dr. F: I don't mean to suggest that you're not bright enough to catch on. Not in the least. What I'm saying is, there are two ways of knowing, from my point of view. First, there is knowing something intellectually. Second, there is knowing something in the heart. Sometimes words aren't enough to help the heart understand.

This equally abstract statement seemed to satisfy the patient. The therapist, though, was wondering if he was capable at this point of extricating himself from a projective identification process in which he had become didactic and pedantic.

Dr. F: I think that your exclusive focus on others' reactions to you causes you to lose your inner voice. When you hear that voice, you'll do better. Until then, you'll be at the mercy of external circumstances.

In this vignette Dr. F felt falsely accused and began to defend himself. By focusing on the patient's extreme sensitivity and the various reasons why blinking might occur, he simply inflamed the situation further. The patient became even more enraged as a result of not feeling understood. Dr. F was focusing on Ms. U's *internal* need to rearrange the external world at the very moment she most needed to externalize. In so doing, he was failing to serve as a container for the bad object and the associated negative affects that she needed to disavow projectively. He then fell into a countertransference need to lecture her, using psychological terms as a way of trying to gain ideational control over the intense affect. Neither strategy particularly helped.

Dr. F's situation is emblematic of a recurrent countertransference issue in the psychotherapy of borderline patients. Therapists must be willing to serve as containers for the bad object projections of the patient (Epstein 1979; Gabbard 1991). Ms. U experienced Dr. F's zealous interpretive approach as trying to force the projection back down her throat. Epstein made the following observation: "The act of interpreting at such moments, then, may be an *unwitting acting out* of our need both to rid ourselves of the unwanted projections and to attack the patient for what he is doing to us" (p. 391). A more useful strategy in such situations is for therapists to contain the projections and to restrict the focus of comments on themselves rather than on the patient. When therapists ask for elaboration on how they are perceived, they do not challenge the patient's perception or interpret that perception as a projection. With this approach the therapist empathizes with the patient's need to deal with strong affects and distressing object-representations by splitting and projective disavowal. The patients will only view the therapist's interpretations as attacks from a "bad object." By asking for elaborations from the patient and not responding defensively, the therapist indicates that the patient's perceptions are taken seriously.

The desirability of containing such projections should not be held up as an unrealistic standard of therapeutic comportment that torments therapists because they rarely feel they can live up to the ideal. All therapists of borderline patients will encounter situations when they feel that the container is overflowing, so to speak, and that their countertransference anger is clear to the patient, as vividly conveyed in the following incident:

> *Ms. T* [arriving 5 minutes late for her session]: Wipe that look off your face! I'm furious at you for not helping me. You do nothing but sit there and listen. Of all the therapists I've had, you're the most worthless!

> At this moment she knocked over an ashtray in which she had placed her cigarette and watched passively as the cigarette proceeded to burn a hole in the therapist's carpet. Dr. G felt himself becoming increasingly enraged at Ms. T to the point where he actually had a visual image of slamming her down on the floor and rubbing her nose in the cigarette burn. He found himself remembering a time when he was 12 years old and physically attacked another boy who was torturing an animal. Dr. G realized that he was being tortured in a similar manner by Ms. T. He actually felt as though he were being physically assaulted. The carpet that was smoldering in front of his eyes was a prized, expensive Oriental rug. He was physically trembling as he attempted to control his voice when he finally spoke.

> *Dr. G:* You will repair that carpet, and you will never smoke in this office again.
> *Ms. T:* You're angry, aren't you?

Dr. G: Yes, what you did made me very angry.

Dr. G's insistence that Ms. T repair the damage she had done and the direct expression of his anger caused Ms. T to become rapidly subdued. But Dr. G soon learned that he had made a mistake to ask his patient to repair the carpet. At the beginning of the next session, she came in with a single-edged razor blade. She immediately knelt down by the carpet and proceeded to cut a hole twice as large as the original hole with the razor blade.

Ms. T: You asked me to repair this, so I'm doing as I was told.

As Dr. G watched in horror, he felt a tremendous sense of despair, as though the situation was hopeless and could not possibly change. He then felt a sense of resignation as his body relaxed. He started feeling more objective about the patient, realizing that she was disturbed and that he could do nothing about the hole that she had made in the carpet. He then proceeded with the session. After the session, however, he felt his anger returning, and he realized that his reaction of becoming calm, objective, and understanding had simply been a defense against the murderous rage he was really feeling.

As we noted in Chapter 4, sometimes we must *react* before we can begin to *respond*. The more we work with a particular patient, the less likely we are to be provoked by predictable patterns of the externalization of an internal object relationship. However, therapists all have their own limits. The rage of borderline patients will eventually get under the therapist's skin. In such circumstances the patient can benefit by seeing the therapist's anger. Trying to disguise or deny the anger may be worse than sharing it with the patient. Especially in the treatment of severely destructive hospitalized patients, both hospital staff members and psychotherapists must feel comfortable in setting limits on certain kinds of affective expression.

Allowing such patients license to hurl racial and ethnic slurs, shout obscenities, and treat everyone with contempt breeds a form of entitlement that is antitherapeutic. Setting limits on what will be tolerated helps patients face the reality that they cannot freely ventilate their feelings toward others without severe consequences. If no limits are set, patients may assume that their treaters feel that expressing their rage is therapeutic and helpful. Hospitalized borderline patients commonly demand that staff members tolerate verbal abuse. They often state that they are in treatment to "get their anger out." In such instances, the treatment staff may need to help patients see that treatment is designed for them to gain control over angry feelings rather than to ventilate them freely.

One study of the therapeutic alliance in the psychotherapy of borderline patients (Frank 1992) indicated that certain hostile reactions by the therapist may even help the patient work more effectively in therapy. In studying the first 6 months of psychotherapy with borderline patients, Frank found an unexpected correlation between therapists' perceptions that they were making negative contributions to the therapeutic alliance and symptomatic improvement in the patient. Frank reflected on some of the therapists' behaviors, including

> the therapist's being overly active and directive; exclusively pursuing his/her own agenda in the session; being critical of the patient; displaying intolerance of the patient's need to perpetuate problems; and conveying disappointment, annoyance, or frustration because the patient was not making sufficient progress. For some patients, these actions may indeed impede the formation of a good alliance and have a negative impact on outcome. For hospitalized borderline patients, these same interventions may be just what is needed to limit regressions, anchor the patients in reality, make maladaptive behaviors ungratifying, and otherwise enable a solid alliance to evolve and structural change to occur. (pp. 237–238)

The central point to be stressed in this discussion is not that therapists should freely ventilate anger at their patients. Rather, they should simply accept that frustration, annoyance, irritation, and sometimes outright hostility will exceed the therapist's ability to contain. At those moments, all is not lost—even behaviors that seem like technical errors may ultimately be useful in helping patients see the impact they have on others and in helping them re-own affective states that they expect others to bear.

Rage Versus Hatred

The role of the aggressive drive is central to both rage and hatred, but the two can be differentiated because hatred is a more stable and enduring affective experience that requires an internal object-representation (Galdston 1987; Pao 1965). Whereas rage may be ventilated against any frustrating external object in the environment, hatred is much more specific. To hate is to hold on to an internal object in an unforgiving way. There is no getting beyond the wish for vengeance, the wish to destroy the object. As Galdston (1987) noted: "The patient cannot get over it alone because hatred binds him to an object from the past in the grip of an ancient grudge that requires transference for its release" (p. 375).

Borderline patients, by definition, have not been able to integrate the loving and hateful representations of others into an ambivalently regarded whole object. Feelings of hate are more likely to appear, then, in a more direct and unmodified form. In fact, there is a subtype of chronically hateful borderline patients whose very essence appears to involve hating those who are in the role of helper. These patients have established a dominant part-object relationship between a hated object-representation and a hating self-representation (Gabbard 1989b, 1991).

These patients often seem to be consumed with venomous contempt because the good, loving aspects of the self and the corresponding object-representations are buried deep within to prevent their destruction by the all-consuming hate. Alternatively, they may be projected into persons in the environment who are regarded as entirely good or totally loving (Boyer 1983; Giovacchini 1975; Hamilton 1986; Klein 1946/1975; Searles 1958/1965). In this manner the islands of love and concern for others are further protected by safely storing them in others. This strategy may well backfire, however, because the perception that others are saintly may produce profound envy. This development may lead the patient to project devalued and hated self- and object-representations as a way of "smearing" the saintly person with undesirable aspects in the patient's internal world (Poggi and Ganzarain 1983).

Benign Versus Malignant
Transference Hate

Transference hate is not a monolithic entity. It varies greatly in intensity, depending on the ego strength and internal object relations of the patient. An analogy may be drawn to Blum's (1973) distinction between erotic and erotized transference. *Erotic* transference is experienced as an ego-dystonic and perhaps shameful feeling of desire for the therapist, the gratification of which is viewed as unrealistic. In *erotized* transference, the patient's observing ego is nowhere in evidence. The longings for the therapist are not viewed as feelings to be analyzed. On the contrary, they form the basis of an ego-syntonic demand for gratification of the wishes with the expectation that the therapist should reciprocate instead of interpret.

If the same distinction is applied to transference hate, we may identify two broad categories (Gabbard 1991). In the more benign variety, the patient recognizes the hate as a distortion requiring exploration and understanding. The hateful feelings are ego-dystonic, so the patient maintains a therapeutic alliance with the therapist in pursuit of understanding the feelings rather than acting on them. In the malignant variant, the "as if" quality to the feelings disappears, and the patient feels that no distortion is involved. The therapist is not viewed as *like* someone from the patient's past, but rather as a truly malevolent individual deserving of hatred. A therapeutic alliance is difficult to establish in such instances, and understanding is viewed as irrelevant.

As a general rule, the benign form of transference hate, like its erotic counterpart, is more characteristic of neurotically organized patients, whereas the malignant variant, much like erotized transference, is more likely to be found in borderline patients (Gabbard 1991). The emergence of this malignant form of transference hate in borderline patients is directly related to their being stuck in the paranoid-schizoid mode of psychological functioning. As noted in Chapter 2, this mode creates extraordinary difficulties for the therapist because the potential space (Winnicott 1971) or analytic space (Ogden 1986) so crucial for the development of a reflective, exploratory stance in psychotherapy has collapsed. The transference hate in these patients lacks the "stand in" or "as if" quality that is viewed by the neurotically organized patient as a current-day repetition of a past relationship. Instead, the patient views the therapist as the *original* object of hate and takes no reflective distance with regard to the perception of the therapist.

Malignant transference hate elicits problematic countertransference reactions in a therapist who is prepared to be viewed as helpful and caring. Managing the feelings provoked by such patients begins with understanding the role that hate plays in the psychological equilibrium of these patients. This subgroup of chronically hateful borderline patients seems to seek out treatment because the very core of their being depends on having a libidinal relationship to attack (Rosenfeld 1987). Kernberg (1984) noted that patients such as these, who are part of a larger group prone to negative therapeutic reactions, are often identified with a cruel, sadistic internal object that can only give some semblance of love if it is accompanied by hatred and suffering. In other words, attachment must always come at the expense of hatred. The alternative is a state of nonexistence.

Therapists who treat hateful borderline patients should remind themselves periodically of the developmental value of hate. As Winnicott (1949) was fond of noting, love and hate are the yin and yang of early infantile experience. One cannot exist without the other. We are unable to reach a state of love if we have not also been able to hate. In addition, several authors (Epstein 1977; Little 1966; Pao 1965) observed that hate serves the function of organizing the ego. Hate may fend off feelings of disintegration, provide a reason to live, and give a sense of continuity from day to day. Hate may serve to shore up boundaries between the patient and therapist when the patient feels threatened by merger.

Containment

The principles of containment outlined in Chapter 4 are certainly applicable to the management of countertransference with hateful borderline patients. Numerous authors (Boyer 1986, 1989; Buie and Adler 1982; Carpy 1989; Chessick 1977; Epstein 1979; Gabbard 1989a, 1989b; Giovacchini 1975; Grotstein 1982; Little 1966; Searles 1986; Sherby 1989) focused on the centrality of containment in the treatment of borderline patients. These authors all agree that 1) verbal interpretations will fall on deaf ears when the borderline patient is harboring intense negative feelings toward the therapist, 2) a new set of experiences with a new object is necessary before the borderline patient can accept interpretive interventions, and 3) the traditional role of the therapist as a neutral observer who delivers occasional interpretations from a position of evenly suspended attention is not an adequate characterization of the requirements for the psychoanalytic treatment of borderline patients.

Although containment is essential to handle hateful feelings generated in the patient-therapist dyad effectively, this strategy is difficult to sustain because powerful feelings of hatred, by their nature, impel us to action, rather than reflection (Heimann 1950). The action chosen may include the use of interpretation as a weapon of counterattack—an attempt to suppress the patient's hostility. These interpretations are also frequently an attempt to unload the hateful self- or object-representation projected into the therapist.

As we noted earlier in this chapter, however, regarding the need to be the container of rage for the rageful patient, returning the projected parts of the hateful patient prematurely via interpretation is usually an error of technique (Carpy 1989; Epstein 1977, 1979; Gabbard 1991; Grotstein 1982; Ogden 1982, 1986; Rosenfeld 1987; Searles 1986; Sherby 1989). Hateful borderline patients need to keep the hateful self- or object-representation in the therapist because these patients are unable to integrate hateful aspects within themselves. Moreover, if therapists cannot tolerate the transference role assigned to them because the projected introject is unpleasant, how can they reasonably expect the patient to tolerate it? Searles (1986) warned that forcing the introject back into the patient through premature interpretation implies a denial of any basis in reality for the patient's transference perception of the therapist. The therapist appears to be telling the patient, "Hate resides only in you, not in me."

Other compelling reasons to avoid premature interpretation of projected aspects of the patient are worth consideration. Unless the therapist has sat with the projected material and subjected it to the metabolizing, detoxifying process of containment (Bion 1962), the therapist will be returning it in the same form in which it was delivered. In its most extreme form, this variant of countertransference acting out may be as dramatic as the case of the young therapist described by Altschul (1979), who grew so exasperated at his borderline patient that he screamed, "I hate you," over the telephone. Although such eruptions of "countertransference psychosis" by a psychotherapist may seem unusual, they occur with some regularity among hospital staff who treat borderline patients. In these cases, the treater has been taken over by the patient's projection, and the patient's inability to integrate good and bad elements of self and object are re-created in the clinician (Altschul 1979). In the moment of countertransference acting out, the therapist, like the patient, sees action—extrusion or destruction of the "bad object"—as the only solution to the intolerable feelings of hatred.

A Case Example

An extended case example illustrates some of these themes.

> Mr. S, a high-level borderline patient, began seeing Dr. H in four-times weekly psychoanalysis after his previous analyst had left town. He began the analysis with almost immediate feelings of contempt toward Dr. H.

> *Mr. S:* I know you think I'm assaultive, but it's because of the way you treat me. You charge me, you even bill me when I choose to take vacations, you don't give me answers to any of my questions, and you rigidly enforce the end of the hour even if I'm in the middle of a thought. I see *you* as assaultive, so I react with hostility.

> Mr. S reacted with scorn when Dr. H would suggest that much of the venom Mr. S directed toward Dr. H was a displacement that actually belonged with the memory of his last analyst. Mr. S sug-

gested that Dr. H was trying to "pass the buck" to someone else for his own failings.

Dr. H felt that Mr. S had a point. Mr. S had indeed been tuning in to Dr. H's attempt to sidestep the heat of the transference by deflecting it elsewhere. Dr. H had grown increasingly frustrated with the absence of analytic space in which the two of them could look at what was being re-created in the transference as a repetition of past relationships. Confronted with no gateway to forging a viable working relationship with the patient, Dr. H was attempting to develop an alliance by encouraging Mr. S to direct his wrath elsewhere. If Dr. H had succeeded, he could have empathized with the hatred Mr. S was feeling toward his previous analyst and, in so doing, could have formed an alliance around the shared anger toward an "outside enemy."

Dr. H's primary reaction to Mr. S's intense hatred was to feel falsely accused because the anger did not belong to him. He occasionally felt some relief when his patient would regard him briefly as an idealized object, but this turn of events led Mr. S to hate Dr. H all the more because envy then emerged.

Mr. S: I see all your books on those shelves, and I feel a sense of loathing toward you. I could never read that many books. I can't ever hope to have the amount of knowledge that you have. I feel like getting up and tearing down all your bookshelves.

Mr. S often would pound his fist lightly on the wall adjacent to the couch as he railed against Dr. H. He would exert some control over the pounding so that it would stop just short of being a disturbance to the occupant of the office next door. Dr. H could never be certain, however, and Mr. S's behavior placed his analyst in a disturbing dilemma. If Dr. H did nothing about the pounding, he felt like he was colluding with this "acting in" by allowing Mr. S to disturb his neighbor. If, on the other hand, Dr. H told Mr. S to stop the pounding, he worried that he would be allowing himself to be manipulated by his patient into a nonanalytic posture in which Mr. S could then rightly view Dr. H as attempting to control him. This was only one of many dilemmas Mr. S presented when Dr. H felt damned if he did and damned if he didn't.

Mr. S would repeatedly try to maneuver Dr. H into a corner

where the analyst would wittingly or unwittingly imply that he
hated the patient. The barrage of contempt day in and day out
took its toll on Dr. H, and he was not always able to contain the
patient's projected contents adequately. Dr. H would occasionally
make sarcastic, contemptuous, or counterattacking comments as
he sought to survive in the lion's den that Mr. S had created in his
office. On one particular day Mr. S accused Dr. H of not empathiz-
ing with his point of view. Dr. H responded with some exasperation
in his voice.

Dr. H: You treat me with contempt and then expect me to empa-
    thize with you. I wonder if this is part of a larger pattern of
    expecting others to love you and take your side without earn-
    ing their regard.
Mr. S: So you *do* hate me. I knew I could get you to admit it.

On another occasion the following exchange occurred:

Mr. S: I don't understand why you give me no credit whatsoever
    for being able to hate you. Don't I get two points for expressing
    my anger?
Dr. H: What do you see as positive about that?
Mr. S: Because all my life I've suppressed my anger. Now I'm fi-
    nally getting it off my chest.
Dr. H: You're speaking of a side of you that I haven't seen. All I
    have seen is unrelenting hostility.
Mr. S: Then you must hate me! You can't handle me! I'm too
    tough! I get a thrill out of triumphing over you and being the
    only patient of yours who will not get better, who won't change
    in the way that you want me to.

Mr. S had made a couple of good points. Indeed, Dr. H did feel
sometimes that he could not handle Mr. S, and he certainly did
hate him at times. One of the most distressing aspects of the analysis for Dr. H was that Mr. S appeared completely uninterested in
receiving help from him. The patient confirmed the accuracy of
this observation when the analyst pointed out to him that he repeatedly defeated any effort on the analyst's part to help him understand himself. Mr. S's response was explosive:

Mr. S: I don't fucking want your help! I want you as a target! I
    attempt to provoke you. I have a fantasy of throwing up on your

floor or shitting on your couch. I want to rid myself of all this.
I hate it when I can't provoke you into taking my anger. Then
I have to take it. I need a place to dump. I've been using you
like a pay toilet.

This outburst helped Dr. H to understand how Mr. S conceptualized the analytic process. It was indeed a toilet. It was a place
where he could evacuate the bad aspects of himself and his tormenting and hated internal objects. From his point of view, projection of these mental contents was a far superior option to any other
alternative. His behavior in the hours made Dr. H feel coerced into
accepting the role of the hated object that hated him back. Dr. H
resorted to numerous defensive maneuvers to avoid the role. At
times he would withdraw and become more aloof, attempting to
retreat into defensive isolation where he would be impervious to
Mr. S's attacks. At other times he would attempt to empathize with
Mr. S's need to hate as a means of emotional survival. In still other
instances, Dr. H would shore up his occupational reaction formation by attempting to feel loving concern for the poor wretch.
When Dr. H would shift into this mode, Mr. S would invariably experience him as being less than genuine, not to mention patroniz-
ing.

Dr. H's countertransference loathing reached a peak when he
had a thorny scheduling problem and asked his patient if he could
change the analytic hour on Wednesdays. Mr. S replied that while
he probably could switch the hour to accommodate Dr. H's wish,
he was choosing not to do so. Mr. S said that it was important for
him to assert his own rights rather than to allow others to "walk
over me." Mr. S went on to say that he experienced tremendous
pleasure to know that he could control Dr. H rather than allowing
his analyst always to be the one in charge. His refusal to cooperate
left Dr. H seething with resentment. Dr. H began to dread having
to see the patient day after day, and he found himself wishing that
Mr. S would quit. Driving home in the evening, Dr. H would find
himself daydreaming about what he might do to make Mr. S decide
to quit. He also imagined "zingers" that he would like to say to
Mr. S, knowing all the time that he could never express direct in-
sults in the analytic hour. However, the fantasies about what he
would like to say helped Dr. H metabolize and bear the intense
hatred that Mr. S evoked in him.

In the midst of this intense countertransference hatred, Dr. H went on a 2-week vacation. As the vacation neared its end, Dr. H found himself dreading his return to work because he would have to face the unpleasant experience of a 50-minute hour with Mr. S each day. On the night before he returned, Dr. H had the following dream: *Mr. S and Dr. H were in an analytic session. Dr. H was growing increasingly anxious as Mr. S continued to pound the wall next to the couch with ever increasing intensity. Quite unexpectedly, he turned around and looked at Dr. H and then stood up from the couch and stared down at his analyst with a defiant grin. Dr. H felt frantic that he was unable to control Mr. S, and he unleashed his pent-up fury in the form of a lecture shouted at the top of his lungs: "Analysis is for people who can control their impulses and channel them into words. If you can't do that here, if you can't cooperate with what I am trying to do, you should not be in analysis."* End of dream.

As Dr. H reflected on his dream in an effort at self-analysis, he thought of the many times when Mr. S pounded on the wall. He had often wanted to say just those words to him. The dream helped Dr. H to understand why he had not. For Dr. H to assert the customary expectations of the analytic setting carried with it a risk. His unconscious concern was that his intense hatred of Mr. S and his sadistic wishes to control his patient, so evident in the dream, would show through his efforts to clarify the nature of their task. He realized that his guilt related to those feelings was leading him to feel "disempowered" as an analyst. In this context he suddenly understood the meaning of his proposal of the hour change on Wednesdays as an *option* rather than as a decision that had already been made with which Mr. S was expected to comply. At an unconscious level, the ordinary power and control inherent in the analytic role was equated with omnipotent control driven by enormous aggression. Hence, Dr. H's presenting the change as a *choice* could be understood as a reaction formation against those powerful wishes within him.

Another insight Dr. H gleaned from the dream was that the patient had been serving as a receptacle for that part of him that desperately needed to control Mr. S. Dr. H could disavow that part of him by thinking it was *Mr. S* who was driven by the wish to control—not Dr. H. His self-analytic work with the dream brought Dr. H in touch with the fact that his analytic "work ego" (Fleming 1961) was being eroded by the intensity of the patient's projec-

tions. He was starting to share Mr. S's propensity to view action—
not understanding—as the solution.

When the analysis resumed after the break, it was clear that the
break had done both patient and analyst some good. Mr. S began
by commenting that he had been worried ever since the ending of
their last session:

Mr. S: I was afraid I'd pushed you into a breakdown where you
would destroy furniture and attack me. I tried to bait you to
take on my characteristics. I hate it when you're calm—then I
have to take it back in me. I feel like I want to explode. I want
to rip up your office. If I can't be your best patient, maybe I can
be your worst. But I'm afraid that I'll drive you crazy.

Dr. H took advantage of this moment of reflectiveness and the
accompanying opening of analytic space and made an interpretation:

Dr. H: The feelings you have inside are unbearable, but if you
dump them into me, you feel that you will get well at the expense of my going crazy. This worries you, because after all,
feelings of hate are not the only feelings you have toward me.
Mr. S: If I don't hate you, I feel like a primordial soup that is waiting to be pulled together. I have no identity. I want you to take
care of me. I have a pretense of being independent and self-
sufficient, but underneath I'm incredibly dependent and
needy. I don't feel comfortable having anyone take care of me.
I feel diffuse, amorphous, like an amoeba. I feel like being sarcastic with others when I start to feel uncomfortably close.

Changes began to occur on both sides of the analyst-patient
dyad. Dr. H recognized his own countertransference need to take
action to control an analytic situation that was getting out of hand.
In part, he was responding to the patient's projective identification, but he also was reacting to his own anxiety in the face of a
situation in which he had very little control and in which he felt
"deskilled" as an analyst because of his guilt feelings related to the
hate he harbored for Mr. S. On the patient's side of the dyad, a
sequestered object relationship involving a concerned self-
representation (with the capacity to love) and a loved object-representation (with the capacity to be hurt) had surfaced. The

patient's perception of Dr. H's anger and hatred at his refusal to change the appointment time possibly prompted the emergence of the other side of him, accompanied by depressive anxieties as the hating and loving sides of him were juxtaposed. Mr. S also was able to acknowledge the organizing effect of hate on his own sense of identity. In its absence, he felt amorphous. Dr. H's interpretive effort to connect the split-off aspects of his patient further enhanced Mr. S's capacity to look at what lay beneath the hate.

As the analysis proceeded, Mr. S continued to operate predominantly in a paranoid-schizoid mode. However, each foray into depressive concerns was usually associated with an opening of analytic space. At these moments, Dr. H would make interpretive connections for the patient that Mr. S could use to develop his reflectiveness further. One example involved the schedule:

Dr. H: I wonder if your reluctance to change the hour was connected with your fear that I would replace you with someone else. When I proposed to change the Wednesday hour, it may have hurt your feelings.

Mr. S [tearfully]: I've never heard you acknowledge my proneness to feel hurt. No one has ever recognized my pain. I think my worst fear of all is that after I terminate, you won't remember me. I have this fantasy of calling you on the phone many years after the analysis, and you're saying that you don't know who I am.

Dr. H: Your hatred of me is important in maintaining connectedness and avoiding feelings of abandonment. As long as you continue to hate me, you know that I won't see you as ready for termination.

In Dr. H's analysis of Mr. S, the analyst's ability to contain the feelings of hatred projected into him was severely challenged. Mr. S developed a "lavoratoric" transference (Rosenfeld 1987) toward Dr. H. In other words, he viewed Dr. H as a toilet into which he would dump the bad and unacceptable parts of himself. Dr. H's wish that Mr. S would quit the analysis was a re-creation of the patient's part-object world within his own mind. Getting rid of the patient seemed to be the only solution to the analyst's tormented internal state. Dr. H's interventions were not particularly effective at that point in the analysis, and there was a kernel of reality in the patient's perception that Dr. H hated him and was having difficulty handling him. As Gorney (1979) noted, when the patient's entire effort is to transform the therapist into a bad object, there may be a real erosion of the therapist's technical competence as he reacts in a role-responsive manner by becoming "bad" in his choice of interventions and their timing.

Both the analytic work ego (Fleming 1961) and the necessary split between the observing and experiencing aspects of the analyst's ego (Kris 1956) are compromised by the powerful projective identification process that accompanies the malignant form of transference hate. Fortunately, the self-analytic work in which Dr. H immersed himself and the actual break in the analysis gave him the necessary distance to get back on track with Mr. S.

The extended case report illustrates two crucial points about the analytic space. First, patients are not the only ones who fluctuate between the paranoid-schizoid and depressive positions. In the throes of projective identification, therapists themselves may lose their own sense of analytic space as they find it deteriorating into a paranoid-schizoid mode of experience in which ill-advised action seems to be the only way of surviving. The second point is that interpretive work will be effective only when both patient and therapist are coexisting in an analytic space—that is, both are functioning in a mode in which reflective distance, therapeutic alliance, and the creation of a psychic reality independent of the perception of external events are possible. It follows from these two critical points that the successful treatment of malignant transference hate in borderline patients involves prolonged periods of containment that gradually allow for interpretation at a frequency determined by the convergence of analytic space in both patient and therapist.

Part of the containment process in the case of Mr. S involved Dr. H's attempt to trace his own defensive maneuvers as he sought to avoid hating the patient. Hate in the patient tends to evoke hate in the therapist (Epstein 1977), but hate also tends to produce denial of hate. As Winnicott (1949) stressed, analysts must not deny that hate actually exists within themselves and that they actually hate their patients. Patients will be able to tolerate their own hate only if the analyst can also hate. In this regard, Dr. H's sarcasm-tinged confrontations of Mr. S, which Dr. H viewed as countertransference-related "mistakes," may have been useful in some way to the patient. In clinical discussions, therapists are often asked if they can treat patients they do not like. A more relevant question in the case of hateful borderline patients is whether therapists can treat patients they do not hate. Epstein (1977) noted that the most frequent error is for the therapist to react to projections of hatred by attempting to be "all good." This deprives the patient of a primary defensive mode, which is to disavow hatred projectively and to see it in the therapist instead of in oneself.

Therapists also should scrutinize the countertransference temptation to collude with the patient's splitting by focusing on only the good or loving aspects of the patient (Kernberg 1984). As described in the treatment of Mr. S, one variant in this defensive posture is to encourage the displacement of hate onto an extratransference figure, so the therapist can develop a therapeutic alliance based on the extrusion of hate and badness from the therapist-patient relationship.

Another defensive operation requiring monitoring during the containment process is the therapist's tendency to act as if the patient's perception is entirely a distortion, leading to a disavowal of all responsibility and a projection into the patient of qualities that actually reside in the therapist as well. A crucial turning point in the analysis of Mr. S was Dr. H's discovery that Mr. S's perception of his analyst as a punitive person invested in asserting omnipotent control over him was not entirely a distortion. On the contrary, this perception resonated with Dr. H's actual wishes to control Mr. S. In this context, Searles (1986) made the following observation:

> It is essential that the analyst become as open as possible to acknowledging to himself that even the patient's most severe psychopathology has some counterpart, perhaps relatively small by comparison but by no means insignificant, in his own *real* personality-functioning. We cannot help the borderline patient, for example, to become well if we are trying unwittingly to use him as the receptacle for our own most deeply unwanted personality compo-

nents, and trying essentially to require him to bear the burden of all the severe psychopathology in the whole relationship. (p. 22)

Therapists must walk a fine line between blasting the patient with their own hatred and denying its very existence. After hatred and anger are processed and metabolized through the containment process, they can be more constructively expressed in a way that is useful to the patient (Epstein 1977; Searles 1986; Sherby 1989). Moreover, the tolerating of intense feelings in and of itself may produce change in the patient (Carpy 1989).

During the months prior to the 2-week break in the analysis of Mr. S, the patient bore witness to Dr. H's numerous struggles to maintain an analytic posture in the context of being used as a toilet for the patient's unacceptable parts. Dr. H's struggles were manifested in his partial acting out by making sarcastic comments periodically, by withdrawing into aloof silences, by feeling guilt-ridden by his reluctance to enforce the schedule change he proposed for fear that he would betray his aggressive feelings, and by attempting to transcend his hatred by assuming a saintly position vis-à-vis the patient. As Carpy (1989) noted, patients' observation of their therapist's attempts to deal with feelings regarded as intolerable makes those feelings somewhat more tolerable and accessible for reintrojection. Projective identification begins as an attempt to destroy links between patients and their feelings because the feelings are unbearable. Observing the therapist's capacity to bear those same feelings restores the linkages. Mr. S, for example, began to "re-own" some of the feelings that he observed in Dr. H with his comment that, "I tried to bait you to take on my characteristics. I hate it when you're calm—then I have to take it back in me."

One other aspect of containment is the message conveyed to the patient that the therapist is a durable, persistent object that is not destroyed by the patient's attacks. Winnicott (1968/1989) stressed that survival means avoiding retaliation, and he specifically cautioned against using interpretation in the midst of the patient's attacks. He viewed interpretive interventions as dangerous under such circumstances and suggested that the therapist would do better to wait until the destructive phase is over, at which point the therapist can discuss with the patient what transpired during the attacks.

The case of Mr. S demonstrates that one often has to go to the brink of despair with hateful borderline patients before a breakthrough occurs. In commenting on destructive patients, Bird (1972) noted: "This dark and ominous time, when both patient and analyst are about ready to call it quits, is, according to my thesis, perhaps the only kind of transference in which the patient's most deeply destructive impulses may be analyzable" (p. 296). Therapists who can contain the feelings of hate for a sufficient time often find that longings for love are concealed by the hateful feelings. Mr. S was finally able to reveal that he had established an intense dependency on his analyst and wished to preserve some form of connectedness to Dr. H through his hating.

Bollas (1987) coined the term *loving hate* to describe "a situation where an individual preserves a relationship by sustaining a passionate negative cathexis of it" (p. 118). In patients in whom this form of hate resides, hate does not exist as the opposite of love but as a substitute for it. Mr. S, for example, lived with a dread of indifference, and only through hate could he coerce objects in his environment into passionate involvement with him. Only then did he feel alive and connected. Other functions of the hate became apparent as well in the analysis of Mr. S, including its organizing effect on his amorphous sense of identity, its role in defending against grief, and its defensive function in the service of dealing with envy.

The Role of Interpretation

In the foregoing discussion on the management of countertransference with hateful borderline patients, we have stressed the role of containment and the postponement of interpretation. If interpretations are employed early on, they will be experienced as a confirmation that the therapist is like everyone else—a persecutor attempting to attack or victimize the patient. The therapist must have some preliminary understanding of the countertransference arising from the interaction by processing the patient's projections. The therapist needs to accomplish the self-healing task necessary to restore a sense of analytic space before interpretation will be effective. Then the therapist must wait for the patient to converge in a similar space where interpretations will be meaningful.

When Mr. S made comments such as, "I hate it when I can't provoke you into taking my anger," or "I tried to bait you to take on my characteristics," he was indicating some opening of analytic space. He was thinking symbolically about what was happening in the analyst-patient relationship—that is, he was distinguishing between symbol and symbolized. When he expressed open concern that he might drive his analyst crazy, he was clearly operating in a depressive mode of mental functioning with its associated anxiety that he might harm someone he had grown to care about. He had begun to think about what he was doing to his analyst in a way that was analogous to the climactic scene in William Friedkin's 1974 classic horror film, *The Exorcist,* when the demon possessing the little girl leaves her and enters the psychiatrist-priest, leading him to plummet to his death. Mr. S felt he could get over his "madness" only at the cost of driving his analyst mad. Carpy (1989), who also advocated the postponement of interpretation, pointed out that patients are capable of using the interpretation only when they can recognize aspects of themselves in the analyst.

When the split-off and sequestered aspect of the patient's self that contains feelings of love and concern finally surfaces, the therapist's task is to reconnect the split parts through interpretation (Gabbard 1989b; Kernberg 1984). Dr. H pointed out to Mr. S, for example, that the patient's hatred coexisted with feelings of concern for his analyst. The integration of the loving and hating aspects of the self will be threatening at first, and the patient will continue to revert back to hate. Repeated working through will help patients eventually to understand the sources of their resistance.

The real challenge in working with hateful borderline patients is to bear the experience of being hated—as well as the experience of hating the patient back—without acting on it. By way of analogy, Winnicott (1949) once observed, "A mother has to be able to tolerate hating her baby without doing anything about it" (p. 74).

Summary

Tolerating expressions of rage and hatred is one of the most difficult aspects of managing countertransference. Hatred is distinguished from rageful affect by its association with an internal object. Therapists must appreciate that patients projectively disavow bad internal objects as a means of ensuring their own survival. If a hated introject is prematurely returned to the patient via interpretation, the patient is likely to experience it as an attack or a persecution. Therapists must be willing to serve as containers for the hated introject until the patient can tolerate its return in modified form. Nevertheless, all therapists have their own limits, and it may be highly therapeutic for therapists at times to admit that they have reached a point when they can no longer tolerate certain forms of abuse by the patient. Setting limits on the patient's venomous attacks may be necessary for the therapist to survive the process and to serve as a durable object for the patient. Hatred often impels the therapist toward ill-advised action rather than reflection. The analytic work ego may be eroded so that the therapist has just as much difficulty as the patient in achieving an analytic space where fantasies of action can be considered and contained rather than impulsively carried out. Countertransference hatred may also be defended against through reaction formation and efforts to be the "all-good" parent, which then backfires by increasing the patient's envy. Interpretation should generally be postponed until the hateful aspects have been sufficiently contained and a sense of analytic space has been restored.

References

Altschul VA: The hateful therapist and the countertransference psychosis. NAPPH Journal 11:15–23, 1979

Bion WR: Learning From Experience. London, Heineman Press, 1962

Bird B: Notes on transference: universal phenomenon and hardest part of analysis. J Am Psychoanal Assoc 20:267–301, 1972

Blum HP: The concept of erotized transference. J Am Psychoanal Assoc 21:61–76, 1973

Bollas C: The Shadow of the Object: Psychoanalysis of the Unthought Known. New York, Columbia University Press, 1987

Boyer LB: The Regressed Patient. New York, Jason Aronson, 1983

Boyer LB: Technical aspects of treating the regressed patient. Contemporary Psychoanalysis 22:25–44, 1986

Boyer LB: Countertransference and technique in working with the regressed patient. Int J Psychoanal 70:701–714, 1989

Buie D, Adler G: The definitive treatment of the borderline patient. International Journal of Psycho-Analytic Psychotherapy 9:51–87, 1982

Carpy DV: Tolerating the countertransference: a mutative process. Int J Psychoanal 70:287–294, 1989

Chessick RD: Intensive Psychotherapy of the Borderline Patient. New York, Jason Aronson, 1977

Epstein L: The therapeutic function of hate in the countertransference. Contemporary Psychoanalysis 13:442–468, 1977

Epstein L: Countertransference with borderline patients, in Countertransference: The Therapist's Contribution to the Therapeutic Situation. Edited by Epstein L, Feiner AH. New York, Jason Aronson, 1979, pp 375–405

Fleming J: What analytic work requires of an analyst: a job analysis. J Am Psychoanal Assoc 9:719–729, 1961

Frank AF: The therapeutic alliances of borderline patients, in Borderline Personality Disorder: Clinical and Empirical Perspectives. Edited by Clarkin JF, Marziali E, Munroe-Blum H. New York, Guilford, 1992, pp 220–247

Gabbard GO: On "doing nothing" in the psychoanalytic treatment of the refractory borderline patient. Int J Psychoanal 70:527–534, 1989a

Gabbard GO: Patients who hate. Psychiatry 52:96–106, 1989b

Gabbard GO: Technical approaches to transference hate in the analysis of borderline patients. Int J Psychoanal 72:625–637, 1991

Galdston R: The longest pleasure: a psychoanalytic study of hatred. Int J Psychoanal 68:371–378, 1987

Giovacchini PL (ed): Tactics and Techniques in Psychoanalytic Therapy, Vol 2: Countertransference. New York, Jason Aronson, 1975

Gorney JE: The negative therapeutic interaction. Contemporary Psychoanalysis 15:288–337, 1979

Grotstein JS: The analysis of a borderline patient, in Technical Factors in the Treatment of the Severely Disturbed Patient. Edited by Giovacchini PL, Boyer LB. New York, Jason Aronson, 1982, pp 261–288

Hamilton NG: Positive projective identification. Int J Psychoanal 67:489–496, 1986

Heimann P: On counter-transference. Int J Psychoanal 31:81–84, 1950

Kernberg OF: Borderline Conditions and Pathological Narcissism. New York, Jason Aronson, 1975

Kernberg OF: Severe Personality Disorders: Psychotherapeutic Strategies. New Haven, CT, Yale University Press, 1984

Klein M: Notes on some schizoid mechanisms (1946), in Envy and Gratitude and Other Works, 1946–1963. New York, Delacorte Press/Seymour Laurence, 1975, pp 1–24

Kris E: On some vicissitudes of insight in psycho-analysis. Int J Psychoanal 37:445–455, 1956

Little M: Transference in borderline states. Int J Psychoanal 47:476–485, 1966

McLaughlin JT: The analyst and the Hippocratic oath. J Am Psychoanal Assoc 9:106–123, 1961

Menninger K: Psychological factors in the choice of medicine as a profession. Bull Menninger Clin 21:51–58, 1957

Ogden TH: Projective Identification and Psychotherapeutic Technique. New York, Jason Aronson, 1982

Ogden TH: The Matrix of the Mind: Object Relations and the Psychoanalytic Dialogue. Northvale, NJ, Jason Aronson, 1986

Pao P-N: The role of hatred in the ego. Psychoanal Q 34:257–264, 1965

Poggi RG, Ganzarain R: Countertransference hate. Bull Menninger Clin 47:15–35, 1983

Rosenfeld H: Impasse and Interpretation: Therapeutic and Anti-Therapeutic Factors in the Psychoanalytic Treatment of Psychotic, Borderline, and Neurotic Patients. London, Tavistock, 1987

Schafer R: Psychoanalytic Interpretation in Rorschach Testing: Theory and Application. New York, Grune & Stratton, 1954

Searles H: Positive feelings in the relationship between the schizophrenic and his mother (1958), in Collected Papers on Schizophrenia and Related Subjects. New York, International Universities Press, 1965, pp 216–253

Searles HF: My Work With Borderline Patients. Northvale, NJ, Jason Aronson, 1986

Sherby LB: Love and hate in the treatment of borderline patients. Contemporary Psychoanalysis 25:574–591, 1989

Winnicott DW: Hate in the counter-transference. Int J Psychoanal 30:69–74, 1949

Winnicott DW: The use of an object and relating through identification (1968), in Psycho-Analytic Exploration. Edited by Winnicott C, Shepherd R, Davis M. Cambridge, MA, Harvard University Press, 1989, pp 218–227

Winnicott DW: Playing and Reality. New York, Basic Books, 1971

CHAPTER 6

Sexual Feelings and Gender Issues

The management of sexual feelings—both the patient's and the therapist's—is one of the greatest challenges in the treatment of borderline patients. Many litigated cases of therapist sexual misconduct involve borderline patients (Gutheil 1989). Hence, a systematic approach to sexualized transference and countertransference is essential for good risk management as well as for clinical effectiveness. Erotic feelings may arise in one member of the therapeutic dyad and not in the other or may emerge in both parties simultaneously. In this chapter we examine both variations.

As we noted in Chapter 3, borderline patients often reveal histories of significant childhood sexual abuse. We know that the risk of adult sexual abuse is considerably higher in those persons who have been abused as children when compared with adults who have no such history (Chu and Dill 1990). Specifically, therapist-patient sex is more likely in patients with histories of childhood sexual abuse (Feldman-Summers and Jones 1984; Kluft 1989). Many of these women grew up with the experience of having fused caring and sexuality in all situations. This background may lead them repeatedly to put themselves in situations of revictimization in an effort to actively master passively expressed trauma (Chu 1992).

Another determinant of this higher risk is intimately related to how borderline patients inspire rescue fantasies in treaters. As discussed in Chapters 1 and 3, in a concerted effort to prove that they are unlike the patient's abusing parents, therapists may find themselves crossing one boundary after another as they descend down the "slippery slope" toward sexual contact with the patient. More-over, therapists are often tempted to foster a positive or idealizing transference to avoid the explosions of rage when the borderline patient is disappointed or "crossed." This idealized "good parent-ing" posture may blend into erotic attraction. Therapists who treat borderline patients must be comfortable with their own aggression in the form of setting limits on the patient and must be prepared as well to withstand the patient's rage when these limits are set.

Yet another determinant of the increased frequency of sexual boundary violations in treating borderline patients is their diffi-culty in distinguishing between the symbolic and the concrete. As discussed in some detail in Chapter 2, in the paranoid-schizoid mode the borderline patient loses the "as if" quality of the transfer-ence as a result of the collapse of analytic space. Rather than seeing sexualized transference feelings as in part real and in part new ad-ditions of old feelings from past relationships, the patient views the feelings as unequivocally real, compelling, and requiring immedi-ate satisfaction. This variant of erotic transference is what we refer to in Chapter 5 as erotized transference (Blum 1973), an ego-syn-tonic, tenacious demand for sexual gratification, which is primarily found in borderline patients and incest victims and may be highly refractory to interpretive interventions. Being the target of an erotized transference may produce a variety of reactions in the ther-apist, one of which is intense anxiety, as in the following clinical example of a female borderline patient with a new female therapist:

> *Ms. R:* I was thinking about how attracted I am to you. I hate to bring it up. But I can't help it. You're so attractive. You have gorgeous eyes and such nice curves. Sitting here, my skin feels warm and alive.
>
> Dr. I was feeling heat also. But it was primarily in response to the anxiety of feeling on the hot seat as the patient continued to rate her physical attributes.
>
> *Ms. R:* It is all very erotic. Don't you feel it? In the air? I really shouldn't be saying these things. What you must think of me. You probably already have a lover—or lovers. You wear that

diamond ring. I bet that you are engaged. Oh—I shouldn't even be talking about all of this.

Indeed, Dr. I wore a diamond solitaire on her right hand, and this ring could be mistaken for an engagement ring. The therapist found the situation intriguing, however, that the patient had chosen to ignore the easily identifiable wedding band and engagement ring that Dr. I wore on her left hand. Dr. I assumed that Ms. R did not want her to be exclusively heterosexual nor sure if she wanted the therapist to be in a committed relationship. Yet, at the same time, the patient needed to invent an engagement.

Dr. I: The thought of my being engaged is a safeguard?
Ms. R: I suppose so. These feelings are stronger than they have ever been before. My skin tingles all over [involuntarily shivering]. I know that you must feel it, too. It's a good thing that you're engaged. I wouldn't be able to resist you if you started talking about how it feels to you.

Dr. I was startled by the sudden shift in the patient's perception of her. Only a few minutes earlier the patient had been trying to seduce her. Now, Ms. R was suggesting her wish, and her fear, that Dr. I would seduce *her.*

Dr. I: You're concerned that *I* will act on your feelings?
Ms. R: I don't know what you'll do. I'm sorry—I have to say this— you're so beautiful. I can't believe how strong these feelings are. I know I've told you before that I thought you had a nice figure. But—well, can't you feel it in the air? God, you're smart, too. It's almost time to go, isn't it? Really, I shouldn't have said anything about how I felt. But I can't explain it. It's churning deep down inside me. Is it warm in here? My skin feels so warm. Will you be able to manage this? Will you be expecting me to do something other than talk next time?
Dr. I: Are you worried that I'll act on your feelings and stop being your therapist?
Ms. R: Yes! Exactly! Do you think you can do it? Still be my therapist with all these feelings in the air? I hope you can manage it. Well, I guess it's time for me to leave now. See you next week.

After Ms. R walked out of the office, Dr. I called her answering service to pick up messages. She then headed to the bathroom out in the hallway next to her office. When entering the bathroom, Dr. I was surprised to see Ms. R at the sink. Ms. R squealed with delight: "Oh! My therapist in the bathroom!" Dr. I offered a rather sickened smile and a slight nod. Since she was several paces into the restroom, she felt it would not be a good idea to turn around and leave. She certainly did not want to give the patient the idea that she was running away from her, although her anxiety was driving her to do exactly that. All Dr. I could think about was Ms. R's fear that Dr. I would try to seduce her. She found herself in a situation that seemed to be the worst possible thing that could have happened on the heels of such a session. Would Ms. R think that Dr. I had followed her into the bathroom?

These concerns raced through Dr. I's mind in a fraction of a second. She concluded that, all things considered, the best plan of action was simply to use the facilities as she had intended to do. Trying not to break her stride perceptibly, she proceeded to the stall farthest away from the sink. Once having locked the door, Dr. I resolved not to leave the stall until she heard Ms. R exit the bathroom. She waited for what seemed like an eternity. From what she could tell, Ms. R slowly washed her hands, then meticulously fixed her hair, and then carefully applied her lipstick. After a painfully long time, Ms. R opened the door and walked out without saying a word. Dr. I rushed to her office to pick up her purse and briefcase before driving to an appointment across town. As she left her building, to her continued chagrin, Ms. R was seated on a bench at the front door smoking a cigarette. Ms. R smiled. Dr. I nodded and hurried past before she could be trapped again.

Although this clinical situation may seem humorous in retrospect, at the time, Dr. I was anxious to the point where she felt completely discombobulated. In Chapter 5 we described the power of malignant transference hate to dislodge therapists from their own analytic space. The same is true of intense feelings of a highly sexualized valence (Gabbard, in press). Dr. I felt that action was her only recourse to deal with what seemed like uncontainable affects. The sense of threat posed by the feelings was accentuated by Ms. R's clear loss of boundaries, as manifested by her concern that *Dr. I,* rather than she, might not be able to manage such feelings.

An erotized transference may feel like an invasion of the

therapist's private space. Containment under such circumstances is an extraordinary challenge. The anxiety generated by the invasiveness—as well as by the unconscious or barely conscious sexual arousal in the therapist—may lead the therapist to withdraw into an aloof remoteness or into a counteroffensive of premature interpretation (Gabbard 1994). The therapist must walk a fine line between appearing to flee from the feelings and appearing to collude in an attempted seduction by encouraging further elaboration of the feelings. When (and if) the patient reenters an analytic space where some reflective distance from the feelings can be taken, the therapist can then assume a more interpretive posture.

In some instances, however, action is indeed the only recourse. The therapist may set limits on the patient in no uncertain terms—a concrete transference occasionally requires a concrete response.

> In the middle of a therapy session, a patient announced to her therapist that she was in love with him. She then stood up, crossed the room, and began to give her therapist a back massage. He told her to please return to her chair. He then offered the following confrontation: "I can only do therapy with you under certain circumstances. One is that you must sit in *that* chair and I must sit in *this* chair. Another is that we must use words instead of touch."

In both examples, the hostility underlying the erotized transferences is apparent. Both patients were putting their therapists in highly uncomfortable situations. The unconscious wish to torment and defeat the therapist often lies just beneath the surface of professions of love. Indeed, the message of an erotized transference is that the therapist's training and technique are worthless—only love (or sex) is helpful. Some borderline patients will engage their therapist in an argument about the therapeutic value of love. A useful clarification in such circumstances is that love indeed may have tremendous therapeutic benefit, but to be effective, that love must come from an appropriate romantic partner, not from the therapist. The therapist's task is to help the patient understand obstacles that occur in intimate relationships, including the transference situation, and then apply that learning to outside relationships.

The Erotized Countertransference

The erotic-erotized distinction applied to transference has its counterpart in the therapist's countertransference. In many cases of sexual misconduct, a form of lovesickness occurs (Gabbard 1991; Twemlow and Gabbard 1989), in which the therapist also loses the "as if" sense of the therapist-patient relationship. Therapists in this state feel that they are truly in love with the patient and that those feelings transcend countertransference considerations. The erotized countertransference is especially common in middle-aged therapists who are in a state of despair, often associated with disruption in their personal lives, such as separation, divorce, or other losses. A young, vibrant, sexually provocative borderline patient may seem like a cure for the therapist's dysphoria.

As we noted in Chapter 3, therapists commonly harbor conscious or unconscious fantasies that love is curative, a belief often mirrored by the patient. In addition, suffering therapists may project their own needy, dependent self into the patient and confuse their own needs with the patient's needs. In this form of folie à deux, both members of the dyad have projected aspects of themselves into the other and behaved as though the other has been magically transformed.

The erotization of the countertransference, in many cases, is preceded by a series of capitulations to the patient's demands for a clear demonstration of caring. A key component in preventing the escalation of the erotization is to set limits early on and to help the patient with two distinct but related tasks: 1) distinguishing the difference between the literal and the symbolic, and 2) mourning the fact that neither the therapist nor anyone else can fully make up for parental failures during childhood.

Casement (1985) discussed a case in which he had to set limits as a way of drawing such a distinction between literal and symbolic holding. His female patient asked him to hold her hand because her mother had always refused. After considering her request over a weekend, he concluded that to acquiesce to his patient's wishes would be a way of bypassing the original trauma. He explained to the patient that she needed to experience the trauma *as it had been* to get over it. The patient became enraged and suicidal. She rebuked him caustically: "You *are* my mother, and you are *not* holding me" (p. 162).

Casement (1985) processed and contained this psychotic projective identification in which he found himself immersed and was finally able to intervene in an interpretive form with the patient. He told her that she was evidently making him feel the same sense of despair that she felt. He said that the only way he could help her was to tolerate what she was making him feel. After considering his comment, the patient replied that she believed him for the first time and said she was amazed that he could bear the feelings that she found unbearable.

Therapeutic Use of Countertransference

As with all countertransference feelings, those involving sexual urges should not be viewed as only an interference with the therapeutic process. These feelings are also sources of valuable information about the patient's internal world. If we seek to suppress sexual stirrings in ourselves, we will also limit our effectiveness as therapists. In the following clinical illustration, the therapist had to struggle with his own reluctance to acknowledge and accept his sexual feelings:

> Ms. Q was seeing Dr. J in twice-weekly supportive-expressive psychotherapy. She was taking the therapy seriously and using it to bring about substantial changes in her life. She never expressed any comment that suggested an erotic transference toward Dr. J and seemed to be able to accept the limitations of the professional relationship.
>
> Nevertheless, she frequently wore very short skirts to the therapy sessions and crossed her legs in such a way that her crotch was exposed to Dr. J at various times in the course of the therapy. Although Dr. J made a concerted effort to listen to the psychological themes she brought to psychotherapy, he noticed sexual feelings toward her creeping into his conscious awareness. He also noticed his eyes drifting downward and had to remind himself to restore

eye contact. These reminders were often accompanied with a tendency to berate himself for allowing his thoughts to wander in the direction of erotic fantasies.

Despite his efforts to suppress his sexual thoughts and reestablish his connection with the material she was bringing to the sessions, he found himself wondering how nice it would have been if he had met his patient under different circumstances. Eventually, Dr. J recognized that he was putting forth considerable effort to banish information from his mind that might be highly significant for the therapeutic process.

As he contained his feelings, he reflected on the possibility that his experience with Ms. Q was similar to that of other men. He also attempted to identify any countertransference issues in the narrow sense: Did she remind him of someone from his past? Was his struggle a repetition of a similar struggle that went on in other situations? After embarking on this self-analytic process and deducing that his reaction probably said as much about Ms. Q as about his own unconscious conflicts, Dr. J decided to make therapeutic use of his countertransference feelings.

At an appropriate moment in the therapy, he commented to Ms. Q that she often sat in such a way that she was exposing herself in a manner that some might consider suggestive. He wondered with her if this issue had ever come up with other people.

After rapidly adjusting her skirt, Ms. Q responded that she really had very few "hang-ups" about her body. She went on to inform Dr. J that she often went sailing with her male friends and took off her top to sunbathe on the deck of the boat. She clarified that there was nothing sexual in this behavior and that it simply reflected how comfortable she felt with her friends.

To this revelation Dr. J asked if the men accompanying her on the boat also viewed her topless sunbathing as nonsexual, or if they perhaps had a different view of it. Ms. Q responded that, in fact, men often misinterpreted her. She said she had wondered for a number of years why men approach her as though she is giving them a "come on." She said that a number of sexual relationships with men began that way. They had assumed she was giving off signals of her sexual availability, and they often attempted to seduce her. She flushed with embarrassment and indicated that she found saying no to be very difficult and frequently went along with the men's advances even when she did not know them well.

Dr. J then asked her if this had been a long-standing pattern and if it reminded her of anything from her past. Ms. Q replied that her self-esteem had always depended on her being a sex object for her father. She was convinced that her father would have nothing to do with her unless she submitted to his sexual overtures. With a good deal of shame she revealed that her father would frequently come into her bedroom at night and fondle her genitals while he told her stories.

Much later in the therapy process, Ms. Q commented on how she had learned to establish boundaries in relationships with men. With considerable poignancy she told Dr. J that psychotherapy had been extremely important to her because for the first time she had felt valued as a person by a man without a sexual relationship being involved.

In this fragment of a psychotherapy process, a therapist allowed himself to experience freely feelings that he was struggling to suppress. By processing his erotic countertransference, he discovered in collaboration with the patient that the feelings were part of a reenactment of the patient's childhood relationship with her father. Being sexually available to her father had become a way of ensuring his continued involvement, and her exposure to her therapist was an unconscious effort to stave off abandonment. She felt that the only way she could be valued was as an object of male sexual desire, so she sat in a way that she unconsciously felt would engage Dr. J and keep him involved with her. The therapeutic use of countertransference in this instance led to an opening up of the patient's incest history that was previously unknown to the therapist.

The Value of Consultation

In Chapter 2 we discussed the value of systematically monitoring deviations from the therapeutic frame as possible indices of countertransference. In the case of erotic or erotized countertransference, one should similarly monitor any tendency to step out of a professional role with the patient. Departures from a professional role may or may not be problematic in any given case, but common countertransference developments that may serve as early warning signs of trouble include the following:

1. Self-disclosure of the therapist's own problems
2. Meticulous concern about one's dress and appearance on the day of therapy with a particular patient
3. Sexualized daydreams or fantasies about the patient between sessions
4. Frequent dreams about a particular patient
5. Rescue fantasies about the patient, such as, "I'll be a better parent than the original parents," or "All this poor woman really needs is the right man—if we had only met under other circumstances!"
6. A feeling of being overwhelmed and anxious in the face of powerful sexualized transference feelings

When one or more of these phenomena take hold, the therapist should seriously consider seeking a consultation with a respected colleague. Chessick (1977) suggested a general strategy of lining up a good consultant before beginning the therapy and making a commitment to oneself that the consultant will be contacted at the first sign of falling in love with the patient. The need for this kind of internal commitment reflects the observation that lovesick therapists often would rather do nothing but bask in the glow of the feelings. Moreover, there is a point of no return in cases of countertransference love, after which the advice of a consultant will fall on deaf ears because lovesickness has the therapist in its grip.

The luster of the patient often vanishes when the therapist and the consultant collaborate in an attempt to understand the countertransference (Chessick 1977). A consultant also serves as an auxiliary ego (and superego) to a therapist whose analytic work ego is temporarily faltering. An objective third party, unfettered by the heat of the patient's transference, can help the therapist think through the multiple meanings of the erotization and the logical consequences of various choices. What is being repeated? Who has the patient become for the therapist? Who has the therapist become for the patient? What would the consequences be if the therapist agreed to start hugging the patient at the end of each session?

The self-destructive and aggressive components of both parties' sexual wishes often become patent when a consultant's help is enlisted. The consultant can help by fostering a spirit of non-judgmental openness. Direct questions about the therapist's countertransference fantasies often are helpful in breaking the ice. Consultees can make the process more productive and useful if they make a concerted effort to share the longings and wishes they would most like to conceal from the consultant.

Specific Gender Issues

The identification of relevant gender issues in the psychotherapy of borderline patients is complicated by the identity diffusion that is a central aspect of the psychopathology (Kernberg 1975). Identity diffusion evokes a lack of clarity about being masculine, feminine, male, female, heterosexual, homosexual, biscxual, or some mixture thereof. Complicating this confusion about one's sexual identity is the frequent presence of polymorphous perverse sexual fantasies or behavior that causes borderline patients to doubt who they are and what they want in terms of sexual gratification. One solution to this lack of certainty is for borderline men and women to adopt an exaggerated caricature of their gender as a defensive posture.

Female borderline patients may have learned that by adopting a dependent and seductive stance vis-à-vis male helpers, they are able to receive the maternal nurturance they crave. Some male therapists may respond to this "damsel in distress" presentation by becoming the "knight in shining armor" who will rescue the patient from her plight. In cases of sexual misconduct in which the rescuing has become overtly sexualized, these therapists are frequently surprised to discover that the sexual relations do not appear to satisfy the patient's longings. In other words, she turns out to be more interested in a breast than a penis.

Because of sex-role stereotypes in the culture, male borderline patients may be highly conflicted about their dependent longings and adopt a hypermasculine swagger to deny their passive wishes.

Female therapists may be sexually attracted to the "macho" characteristics of these patients while simultaneously finding their maternal instincts aroused by the "baby" detectable beneath the swaggering exterior. This peculiar mixture of feelings is often linked to a conscious or unconscious fantasy that the right woman could reform the male patient and get him headed in another direction. Again, by examining the relatively unusual situation of female therapist–male patient sexual misconduct, we get a glimpse of certain countertransference enactments. Many such cases involve a female clinician drawn to a roguish but charming man with a diagnosis of substance abuse and borderline personality disorder. The therapist has been swept off her feet by the man and is convinced that her love will "settle him down" (Gabbard 1991). This conviction is in keeping with a time-honored cultural myth in American literature and film suggesting that the "right woman" can domesticate a "rowdy" man.

In other cases of the female therapist–male patient dyad, another pattern emerges. Person (1985) pointed out that erotic transference in these gender constellations may be displaced onto a woman outside the therapeutic situation while the patient himself resists awareness of the erotic transference. The female therapist, on the other hand, may be experiencing a confusing mixture of pregenital feelings involving maternal wishes as well as genital attraction. Because of her anxiety about her feelings, she may resist the awareness of the sexualization of the therapy as much as the patient, as the following vignette illustrates:

> Mr. P was a 22-year-old borderline patient seeing Dr. K, a 38-year-old female therapist. During the course of psychotherapy, Mr. P never suggested any conscious sexual longings for his therapist, but his behavior revealed the presence of unconscious erotic wishes that he actively resisted. On two occasions, he turned down the picture of his therapist's husband on her desk because he said he did not like to have him looking at him. Twice during sessions he unbuttoned his shirt to show Dr. K the results of his body-building efforts. One time, as he walked to the door at the end of a session, he said to his therapist, "Oh, my God, I almost patted you on the butt when I walked out." When a sensationalized media case

about an alleged sexual relationship between a male patient and a female therapist appeared in the news, Mr. P became outraged at the unethical behavior of that therapist and insisted adamantly to Dr. K that this immoral clinician should be drummed out of the profession.

Mr. P tended to act out his erotic transference by directing it elsewhere. After about a year of psychotherapy, he began hanging out at a bar that was frequented by prostitutes. Dr. K became concerned that her patient might contract AIDS and began to caution him about safe sex. Although Mr. P was not actually engaging in sexual relations with the prostitutes, Dr. K found herself increasingly worried about that possibility. She sought consultation to get another opinion on how active she should be in her pursuit of protecting the patient, and her consultant called the erotic transference-countertransference dynamics to her attention. Dr. K said she could see how her patient was resisting the awareness of erotic transference, but she had been reluctant to interpret what was going on.

As she reflected on her reluctance, she felt that Mr. P would flatly deny his sexual attraction to her and then humiliate her by laughing at her for thinking that she could be a sexual object to him. As she reflected more on this fantasy, she realized that he was constantly talking about the perfect bodies of the prostitutes that he consorted with, and Dr. K began to feel that she was not attractive by comparison. By colluding with the patient's resistance regarding the erotic transference, then, she felt that she was avoiding humiliation and ridicule.

She also noted in herself a tendency to view Mr. P's displays of his muscles as much like a little boy wanting his mother to be proud of him by showing off. Like the patient, Dr. K denied the sexualized aspects of the displays. She preferred to see the behavior as pregenital. Although aspects of the behavior, indeed, were pregenital, the more overt sexual aspects were much more difficult for both parties to bring up in the therapy process.

When both members of the dyad are male, some patients will develop overt homoerotic or "homoerotized" transferences that may create considerable anxiety in the therapist. When these homoerotic longings are systematically explored, they often appear to be related to primitive wishes for mothering and caretaking (Gabbard, in press). Other male patients are frightened by their erotic or dependent wishes activated by a male therapist and become competitive or contemptuous as a way of defending against the regressive pull. They may excessively challenge every comment the therapist makes, evoking feelings of anger and hatred in the therapist, who may miss the underlying dependent wishes below the surface. The detailed clinical vignette involving Mr. S in Chapter 5 illustrates this transference-countertransference paradigm.

When female therapists are treating female patients, idealizing transferences often appear at the onset of treatment. As described in the case of Ms. Y in Chapter 2, the patient may have an immediate expectation that her desperate need to be taken care of by an unconditionally loving mother will finally be gratified. If the wish is concretized into an expressed desire to suck the therapist's breasts, as in the case of Ms. Y, the therapist may be alienated by the homoerotic aspects of the wish. More often, however, the raw, undisguised, and primitive infantile wishes are likely to be responsible for anxiety in the therapist, who may fear that she will be sucked dry by the patient or lose her boundaries in a merger with the patient. The therapist soon learns that the cannibalistic aspects of the patient's oral wishes are related to intense envy of the therapist's capacity to give, of her ability to sustain herself in stable relationships, of her ability to bear children (if she becomes pregnant during the course of the therapy), and often of her ability to work as a successful professional. Hence, envy and rage frequently occur on the heals of the idealization, and the therapist may be the target of the patient's contempt. As Coen (1992) pointed out, the misuse of objects for purposes of gratifying dependency needs often serves to mask enormous aggression and envy.

The Therapist's Pregnancy

In any psychotherapy process a therapist's pregnancy has a significant impact. Women who become pregnant find themselves turning inward, becoming more self-absorbed and less interested in their usual pursuits. Pregnant therapists often worry that they are becoming less invested in their patients and not as empathically attuned to their patients' concerns (Bassen 1988; Bienen 1990; Fenster et al. 1986; Lax 1969; Nadelson et al. 1974; Penn 1986). The therapist's pregnancy cannot be hidden. An aspect of her personal life has intruded itself into the therapy and must be discussed. Maintaining the usual boundaries of the psychotherapy becomes an extraordinary challenge. Almost all therapists find some alteration of their usual position regarding self-disclosure nearly impossible to avoid (Bienen 1990). Most patients are curious about the pregnancy, and borderline patients in particular often seize on the opportunity to transgress the usual therapeutic frame and become more personal with the therapist. Invariably, the real relationship between patient and therapist and a push toward greater openness are intensified (Fenster et al. 1986). Associated with this change in the therapeutic relationship is a countertransference feeling of being invaded by the patient, as though the therapist's personal space is no longer her own.

Although all patients are affected by the therapist's pregnancy, seriously disturbed individuals, such as those with borderline personality disorder, have an especially profound reaction. As Bridges and Smith (1988) stressed, seriously disturbed patients experience the therapist's pregnancy as overwhelming their insufficiently developed ability to contain and articulate intense and primitive emotional states. Therapists sense this difficulty and may experience equally intense countertransference feelings as they struggle with the most effective way to manage the situation. A detailed description in the following vignette of one particular therapist's struggle illustrates some of the typical issues that emerge:

> Dr. L had been seeing Ms. O in expressive-supportive psychotherapy twice a week for about a year when Dr. L became pregnant for the first time. She found herself dreading the patient's reaction to the pregnancy and was preoccupied with how best to break the news to Ms. O. She knew that it would be important for her to tell Ms. O before she screamed out an accusation, "You're pregnant!" Dr. L cringed at the thought that her patient would blast her with

how Dr. L was victimizing her. Ms. O had talked often in the psychotherapy about how she would like to have a baby if she were well. However, she chose not to become pregnant because she feared that she would kill her baby since she would be unable to tolerate its neediness.

Dr. L recalled her patient's musings on this subject and recognized that Ms. O's concerns about her adequacy as a mother resonated slightly with her own worries regarding whether or not she would be able to meet her baby's needs. On the other hand, Ms. O's thoughts that she would have impulses to kill her baby far exceeded anything that Dr. L was aware of in herself. Dr. L had always felt invaded and penetrated by Ms. O, and this fear of having her personal space violated was growing more and more intense as she imagined that Ms. O would do something invasive that would hurt her baby. Dr. L became consciously aware of a wish that Ms. O would quit therapy so that she would not have to deal with the situation at all.

As Dr. L continued to ponder the impact of the pregnancy on Ms. O, she found herself wishing that it were possible simply to avoid discussion of the baby in the therapeutic relationship. In fact, she wanted to say to Ms. O, "Leave the baby out of it!" She wanted to rationalize that the baby was a third party and therefore not involved in the therapeutic dyad. She recognized that Ms. O always tended to put some sort of external object between her therapist and her. She imagined that her patient would drag the baby into the relationship and use it in the same manner. It was as though Ms. O could take the baby out of the therapist and put it between them. It made Dr. L extremely angry to think about the potential abuse of her baby.

Dr. L felt her body changing in new and different ways, and she noted a strong desire to hide the baby from her patient. She began to feel that she would not be as flexible and tolerant of the kind of projective identifications she was used to experiencing with Ms. O because of her need to protect her body and her baby. She had often felt drained at Ms. O's tendency to suck her dry of everything she had to give. Now her breasts were growing bigger than ever before in preparation to feed her baby. She felt a sense of dread about having to deal with Ms. O's tendency to sadistically erotize her milk-giving breasts. She felt that this tendency in Ms. O was some sort of perversion in which she no longer felt willing to participate. She became increasingly aware that her sense of survival in the therapeutic situation was taking on a whole new cast. The primary task of surviving the patient's rage and neediness was complicated because the survival of her unborn child was involved. In her personal life, Dr. L felt a growing sense of protectiveness of herself and her baby. For example, she was more selective about what she ate, how she moved, how she wore her seat belt, and what risks she would take. The anticipated blast from her patient seemed much less tolerable now that she had two persons to worry about.

After discussing her feelings at some length with her supervisor and carefully planning a strategy for announcing the pregnancy, the session finally arrived. She began the hour by telling Ms. O that she had something important to tell her, and she wanted her to promise she would stay put and listen to it. (Ms. O had run out of Dr. L's office in the past when distressed.) Ms. O looked alarmed and afraid. She asked Dr. L if she were about to announce that she was stopping the therapy with her. Dr. L reassured her that this was not her plan and that indeed she had no plans in the future to do anything like that. She went on to say that she was pregnant and her baby was due in approximately 6 months.

Defying Dr. L's expectations, Ms. O responded with relative calm. She told Dr. L that she was lucky to be pregnant. She spontaneously commented, "I want to be both a mother and a baby." Then she went on to say that Dr. L was lucky to be educated, married, a professional woman, and pregnant. Her continued comments on her therapist's luck, of course, involved a way of dealing with her envy. Dr. L pointed out to her that she was casting her therapist in the role of being lucky and herself as unlucky.

As Ms. O's reaction was explored further in the session, she started to think about maybe transferring to another therapist. Dr. L explained that the wish to flee that Ms. O was describing had been the reason Dr. L had prefaced her comment at the beginning of the session by extracting a promise that Ms. O would not leave the office. Dr. L found herself becoming more self-disclosing than usual—she noted that she felt some concern about how good of a mother she would be and worried some about the baby's welfare. Ms. O responded in a reassuring manner: "I'm sure you'll be a very good mother." Dr. L then felt some regret that she had made such a poor intervention without thinking.

After the session was over, Dr. L was struck at how well Ms. O had accepted the news compared with her fantasies of catastrophe. She began to recognize that Ms. O was an ideal container, holding Dr. L's own fantasies and feelings about the pregnancy. In supervision after this session, she recognized that her own aggressive wishes toward the baby could be conveniently disavowed and projected into Ms. O.

After announcing her pregnancy, Dr. L felt increasingly invaded by Ms. O's questions and comments in the next few sessions. Ms. O continued to say that Dr. L was lucky to be having a baby. In one session the patient reflected a bit and noted, "I could never have a girl. I'd be too jealous of her. Especially if my husband or lover were to become attached to her. I'd do better with a boy." Dr. L was puzzled by this comment and asked her what made her think that the baby would be a girl. Ms. O said that she was certain that the baby was a girl based on her "intuition." She explained that she was always 100% accurate in predicting the sex of her friends' babies. Dr. L found her intuitive claim a bit disconcerting. Again, she felt that Ms. O was getting inside of her even though her claim was basically preposterous. She had heard this kind of statement before from others but had been far less bothered by it.

About 2 months later, Ms. O began to ask direct, personal questions about the pregnancy. She asked how old Dr. L was. She asked if her therapist could feel movement. She wanted to know what the baby's name was going to be. She inquired about whether or not Dr. L was fixing up a nursery in her home. She commented that her therapist's belly was growing larger and larger and that it would be huge by the time she was 9 months along. She also asked how it felt when the baby moved.

Dr. L had been prepared for these kinds of questions and tried to answer those that seemed the least personal or intimate. For example, it seemed relatively innocuous to tell her that she was indeed feeling movement. She reasoned that at this stage in her pregnancy, anyone would be feeling movement and to acknowledge that to Ms. O was perfectly acceptable. When her patient commented on the size of her belly, Dr. L felt more uncomfortably self-conscious. Also, she felt strongly that she did not want to discuss the names being considered for the baby. This was a very intimate choice for Dr. L that involved only her husband and herself. She did not want Ms. O involved at any level in that process. Despite having rather general guidelines for herself formulated prior to the session, Dr. L found that Ms. O's curiosity had a certain momentum to it that made her reveal more than she initially had planned, and she ultimately had to set a clear boundary for her patient and stop the questions.

The countertransference struggles described in this vignette are typical of the reactions engendered by a therapist's pregnancy, especially when treating borderline patients. Most therapists feel a strong desire to hide their pregnancy as long as possible, even though they may have a simultaneous wish to tell the world about it (Imber 1990). Lax (1969) related this desire to the fear that the patient will somehow rob the therapist of the baby. Dr. L clearly became consciously aware of such concerns as she thought about when and how she would announce the pregnancy.

Virtually all pregnant therapists find themselves worrying about the baby's safety and struggling with countertransference fears that the patient's anger and sadistic fantasies will hurt the baby (Fenster et al. 1986). After the announcement, Dr. L gained considerable insight into the defensive projection of her aggressive feelings toward the baby and the use of the patient as a container for those feelings. Lax (1969) noted that the therapist's own childhood feelings about the birth of a sibling can be activated by her pregnancy and attributed to the patient as a way of denying the feelings in herself.

Highly charged feelings of negative valence may be warded off during pregnancy as a way of protecting the therapist's internal space (Imber 1990). The therapist's feeling afraid of the patient's aggression, then, may simply be a way of not acknowledging how concerned she is about her own aggression. Winnicott (1949) noted that a mother may have multiple reasons why she would hate her baby before it is ever born. Feelings of hatred and anger are much more disturbing when the therapist is pregnant. As Dr. L noted in herself, greater feelings emerge of needing to survive and protect the infant that result in avoiding difficult internal states, even though they may be essential for the effective management of transference and countertransference issues.

Another dimension of Dr. L's reticence to bring up the pregnancy with Ms. O was her fear of the patient's envy. Many pregnant therapists have reported feelings of guilt in response to stirring up the patient's envy by getting pregnant (Bassen 1988; Fenster et al. 1986; Lax 1969; Penn 1986). Other sources of envy in the therapist's personal life can be kept out of view from the patient, at least to some extent, but the pregnancy is undeniable. Guilt feelings may also arise from concern that she is abandoning her patient so she can take care of her baby.

The surprising response of Ms. O to Dr. L's announcement is not atypical. Bridges and Smith (1988) noted that seriously disturbed patients often verbalize little, if any, reaction to a therapist's pregnancy. However, the authors also stressed that patients may show their reaction through a deterioration in their functioning or an increase in symptomatology. Therapists must avoid colluding with the minimization of the patient's reaction and be attuned to their own wishes to avoid the negative feelings in the patient engendered by the pregnancy. Most borderline patients have a profound longing to be mothered, and often the therapist's pregnancy presents them with a rival with whom they cannot compete. The baby will receive the kind of maternal care from the therapist that the patient can only dream about. The envy and despair aroused by this situation may be so overwhelming that the patient simply cannot articulate them. The feelings may only be expressed behaviorally, and the therapist's task may be to help translate actions into words for the patient.

Male patients may react to their therapist's pregnancy with dismay because at an unconscious level the oedipal situation has been re-created in front of their eyes. A woman they thought belonged to them turns out to belong to someone else. They must struggle with feelings of betrayal, jealousy, disappointment, and rage.

The pregnant therapist may respond to her male patient's reaction with irrational feelings of guilt, as though she actually has betrayed her patient. She may also experience a strange sense of embarrassment related to a feeling that her previously concealed sexual activity has now been openly revealed. The therapist's feelings of guilt and shame may be exacerbated by accusations of male borderline patients that the therapist is irresponsible, "loose," or untrustworthy.

Countertransference feelings during pregnancy will always be problematic. The unique convergence of the personal and the professional has few parallels in the practice of psychotherapy. Several guidelines are helpful in managing the situation.

First, before announcing the pregnancy to the patient, the therapist should have in mind a fairly well-established timetable for maternity leave. She should decide on the amount of time she is taking off work based on *her* needs and those of her family, not on imagined pressures from the patient or guilt feelings derived from those imagined pressures. A colleague should also be lined up for coverage during the absence so that patients do not feel entirely abandoned during the maternity leave. Then at the time of the announcement to one's patients, these details can be presented along with the announcement to help patients deal with their anxiety about the future.

Second, therapists who discover that they are pregnant and experience countertransference anxieties would also do well to consult with a supervisor or a respected colleague. The irrational concerns can be dealt with in this context along with realistic issues of how to set appropriate boundaries with borderline patients during the pregnancy.

Third, pregnant therapists need to think through what they will and will not disclose about themselves to their patients prior to bringing up the pregnancy in psychotherapy. Dr. L noted that a certain momentum builds as one question after another comes at the therapist, and whether to respond or set limits may be difficult to decide during a flurry of questions. Some balance between complete self-disclosure and complete secrecy is probably optimal, but the exact proportion of sharing versus concealment must be an individual decision made by the therapist based on her own sense of comfort. Often a supervisor or colleague can be helpful in deciding which questions should be answered and which should be politely parried.

Fourth, above all, therapists should carefully monitor their own reactions to the pregnancy. Guilt feelings in particular should be noted so that therapists avoid being coerced by angry borderline patients into ill-advised changes in their plans. Because of guilt feelings, some therapists end up disclosing more than they had wanted or even changing their maternity leave plans. Some therapists have agreed to regular phone calls during the maternity leave, only to later regret the intrusion into their first few weeks at home from the hospital. All psychotherapists, even those who will never be pregnant, must resolve within themselves that they will not lead their lives in a manner that is designed to please their patients. We all must design our lives to meet the needs of our loved ones and of ourselves, and patients must adjust to those choices.

Summary

Borderline patients, many of whom are victims of childhood sexual abuse, often develop erotized transferences in which they demand sexual gratification. Many of them grew up with the experience of having fused caring and sexuality in all situations and therefore have no understanding of generational boundaries. Therapists may respond in kind by feeling intense sexual arousal or by reacting with intense anxiety to sexual demands that the patient does not see as requiring reflection or contemplation. In some cases, the therapist must be direct and set clear, concrete limits when verbal interventions are to no avail. When the "as if" nature of the countertransference begins to disappear, therapists must strive to restore their observing capacity and help these patients understand that the feelings they are attempting to evoke in the therapist have a history with past object relationships. When therapists feel overwhelmed by sexual feelings and find themselves actively dreaming and daydreaming about their patient, they should seek consultation with a trusted colleague.

Gender roles in borderline patients are complicated by identity diffusion. Patients may adopt a caricature of sex-role stereotypes in a defensive effort to establish their gender or may demonstrate considerable gender ambiguity. Genitalization of the transference and countertransference may also serve as a defensive attempt to maintain an organized view of gender and boundaries to resist more primitive urges to fuse or merge. When a therapist becomes pregnant, borderline patients may experience the pregnancy in a devastatingly personal way. They may seize the opportunity to transgress professional boundaries and attempt to develop a more personal relationship with the therapist. They also may experience rage related to intense sibling and oedipal rivalry. Therapists, in turn, may become anxious that the baby will somehow be damaged by the patient's sadistic fantasies in the transference. Efforts to ward off aggression in the therapist-patient dyad may become prominent, and the therapist may find herself feeling guilty about what she has inflicted on her patient. She needs to give careful thought to deciding when and how to tell the patient that she is pregnant.

References

Bassen CR: The impact of the analyst's pregnancy on the course of analysis. Psychoanalytic Inquiry 2:280–298, 1988

Bienen M: The pregnant therapist: countertransference dilemmas and willingness to explore transference material. Psychotherapy 27:607–612, 1990

Blum HP: The concept of erotized transference. J Am Psychoanal Assoc 21:61–76, 1973

Bridges NA, Smith JM: The pregnant therapist and the seriously disturbed patient: managing long-term psychotherapeutic treatment. Psychiatry 51:104–109, 1988

Casement P: On Learning From the Patient. London, Tavistock, 1985

Chessick RD: Intensive Psychotherapy of the Borderline Patient. New York, Jason Aronson, 1977

Chu JA: The revictimization of adult women with histories of childhood abuse. Journal of Psychotherapy Practice and Research 1:259–269, 1992

Chu JA, Dill DL: Dissociative symptoms in relation to childhood physical and sexual abuse. Am J Psychiatry 149:887–892, 1990

Coen SJ: The Misuse of Persons: Analyzing Pathological Dependency. Hillsdale, NJ, Analytic Press, 1992

Feldman-Summers S, Jones G: Psychological impacts of sexual contact between therapists or other health care practitioners and their clients. J Consult Clin Psychol 52:1054–1061, 1984

Fenster S, Phillips SB, Rapoport ERG: The Therapist's Pregnancy: Intrusion in the Analytic Space. Hillsdale, NJ, Analytic Press, 1986

Gabbard GO: Psychodynamics of sexual boundary violations. Psychiatric Annals 21:651–655, 1991

Gabbard GO: Psychodynamic Psychiatry in Clinical Practice: The DSM-IV Edition. Washington, DC, American Psychiatric Press, 1994

Gabbard GO: On love and lust in erotic transference. J Am Psychoanal Assoc (in press)

Gutheil TG: Borderline personality disorder, boundary violations, and patient-therapist sex: medicolegal pitfalls. Am J Psychiatry 146:597–602, 1989

Imber RR: The avoidance of countertransference awareness in a pregnant analyst. Contemporary Psychoanalysis 26:223–236, 1990

Kernberg OF: Borderline Conditions and Pathological Narcissism. New York, Jason Aronson, 1975

Kluft RP: Treating the patient who has been sexually exploited by a previous therapist. Psychiatr Clin North Am 12:483–500, 1989

Lax R: Some considerations about transference and countertransference manifestations evoked by the analyst's pregnancy. Int J Psychoanal 50:363–372, 1969

Nadelson E, Notman M, Arons E, et al: The pregnant therapist. Am J Psychiatry 131:1107–1111, 1974

Penn LS: The pregnant therapist: transference and countertransference issues, in Psychoanalysis and Women: Contemporary Reappraisals. Edited by Alpert J. Hillsdale, NJ, Analytic Press, 1986, pp 287–316

Person ES: The erotic transference in women and in men: differences and consequences. J Am Acad Psychoanal 13:159–180, 1985

Twemlow SW, Gabbard GO: The lovesick therapist, in Sexual Exploitation in Professional Relationships. Edited by Gabbard GO. Washington, DC, American Psychiatric Press, 1989, pp 71–87

Winnicott DW: Hate in the counter-transference. Int J Psychoanal 30:69–74, 1949

CHAPTER 7

Use of Therapist Self-Disclosure

T he issue of therapist self-disclosure raises a variety of thorny dilemmas. Certainly, the therapist is not a cipher. Pictures in the therapist's office, choices of art and other office decorations, books visible on the therapist's desk, and general knowledge about the therapist in the mental health community provide the patient with considerable information. In classical technique, as applied to neurotic patients, such forms of self-disclosure would be the limits of the therapist's self-revelations to the patient. However, just as neutrality does not apply in the same way to borderline patients as it does to neurotic patients, self-disclosure requires a different set of guidelines when working with disturbed patients. A genuine honesty about feelings in the here-and-now may be essential to develop and to maintain a therapeutic alliance with the patient.

We are here advocating limited therapist self-disclosure that is designed to inform the patient of the interpersonal and intrapsychic use that the patient is making of the therapist. The need for this form of countertransference disclosure can be narrowly defined as *clinical honesty* that focuses on the therapist's experience of the patient's impact in the here-and-now moment of the session. Many patients do not experience themselves as "real." They may gain a sense of the real impact that they have on others when the therapist uses self-disclosure.

This form of self-disclosure must be distinguished from a more pervasive type in which therapists actually share their own personal problems with the patient. Certain borderline patients will virtually

143

demand reciprocal problem sharing because of their insistence that no therapist could understand them unless the therapist had suffered in the same way as they had. When therapists allow themselves to be bullied into this type of transference gratification, they have become involved in a boundary transgression that typically leads to further violations of the therapeutic frame that are ultimately destructive to the process (Gutheil and Gabbard 1993). The following clinical vignette illustrates the form of self-disclosure that we feel is useful in the therapy of borderline patients.

> *Ms. N:* I FEEL LIKE HELL!!! I'm not going to waste time. I am very upset. I can't believe how bad this is. I'm not getting any better. I don't have any friends. That's a joke. I'm just too upset to be expected to be able to deal with people. I might as well die. I'm so angry with everyone I know. The people at work! I'm not getting any better. When I enter the "black hole," everyone leaves me alone. They just disappear. I can't describe it . . . it feels like hell!!! Everyone . . . they tell me, "You can get it together." It's not fair! It repeats what has happened to me all my life. When I'd get angry, my mother would disappear. She just wouldn't be available.
>
> *Dr. M* [interrupting]: Two possibilities occur to me, and I can't tell which may be more helpful to you. The first is to ask you to tell me what happened that is so distressing. The second, does it feel like I sent you away? Are you telling me something about how you experience our relationship by talking about these others?
>
> *Ms. N:* I don't know. No! I feel *nothing* for you. This isn't working. This therapy will never work. You don't understand! I might as well kill myself.

The patient's assertion that she felt "nothing" toward her female therapist had been made repeatedly in the 4 months since they had begun. Ms. N's denial of transference had been increasingly accompanied by an apparent poverty of countertransference reactions. During the first half of these sessions, Dr. M typically felt nothing while Ms. N dramatically recounted distressing episodes in her life. However, by the second half of the sessions, feelings of anger and impotence emerged into Dr. M's awareness.

Once again the therapist was impressed by the absence of any feelings in response to the patient's fireworks. Dr. M considered the declaration of suicidal wishes, but could not muster any particular reaction as Ms. N's words became louder and more emphatic. Instead, the therapist thought, "I feel nothing. We have about 40 minutes to go. This affective storm could blow over, but it's too soon to tell. Maybe there is something I can do to decrease its intensity."

Ms. N: My support group doesn't want to listen to me! The more upset I get, the more they are repulsed by me, the more they leave me alone.

Dr. M   [consciously trying to behave differently from the disappointing support group members]: What happened to upset you so?

Although she continued to feel nothing in response to the patient's complaints about disappointing "helpers," Dr. M's notes summarizing the session suggested otherwise. Without realizing her slip, the therapist quoted herself as saying, "Does it feel like I don't want *me* to tell *you* about *my pain?*" A powerful emotional dialogue was transpiring between the patient and the therapist, despite the twin denials of conscious transference and countertransference feelings. Ms. N reassured Dr. M that, in contrast to everyone else in her life, Dr. M was willing to listen. Yet, instead of moving on to discuss the problem at hand as Dr. M anticipated, the patient returned to her droning complaints.

Dr. M   [interrupting]: You say how desperate, alone, and angry you feel when no one asks, yet I've asked a number of times and you don't tell me .

Ms. N: You're right. You are trying. I just wasn't listening. The words that you say disappear inside me. They're gone. I'm sure you meant well. Clearly, my rage and envy destroyed everything that you tried to say. That's what my last therapist used to tell me anyway. He was a brilliant man.

At this point in the session Dr. M's experience of nothing began to shift to a sense of inadequacy, frustration, and annoyance.

Ms. N   [volunteering]: I'm not angry or jealous or dependent on you, because I have no feelings toward you at all. I'm not feeling anything! This isn't working!! I might as well be dead.

Some support group they are! I go and I tell them that I've lost my feelings, and does one person ask me what happened? I can't stand women. I'm *terrified* of women.

Dr. M: You've said before that these outside relationships can tell us something about how you feel in here about our relationship.

Ms. N: I know I said that. But I feel nothing.

Dr. M offered a variety of comments in an effort to provide momentum for a discussion. The patient nicely and intellectually acknowledged the possible relevance of some of her remarks, but Ms. N did not allow any emotional truth to emerge or to be acknowledged. Ms. N reasoned that, since no meaning existed in the therapeutic relationship, no help would be forthcoming. She stated that she might as well kill herself. Having concluded that her suicide was inevitable, Ms. N became increasingly distraught. Soon she was gasping for air because she was crying so hard. Between gasps, she spoke in broken sentences.

Ms. N [tearfully]: I'm [gasp] just [gasp] an innocent [gasp] baby [gasp] who wants to be cuddled [gasp] by a loving mother! [gasp] I want to [gasp] be loved [gasp] but the mother [gasp] doesn't care [gasp] how I feel! I FEEL LIKE HELL!!!

Dr. M became anxious in response to the patient's compelling tears and increasingly loud speech, so she made an attempt to say something empathic to the patient. As before, Ms. N's affective agitation and rageful despair continued. Dr. M, losing faith in the ability of words to affect the course of the session, began to wave her hands to call a time out.

Dr. M: You need to calm down. Take a few deep breaths. [Ms. N began to comply.] You're showing me that you're upset. I can see that you feel like hell. But, you're leaving me in the dark because you aren't using words. You need to slow down so you can use words.

Ms. N [The patient settled gradually and looked around the office. Dr. M also relaxed.]: I want to destroy your office and everything in it.

The steely glare with which the patient delivered her threat to destroy the office came as a surprise. Dr. M's heart sank. She quickly appraised the situation. First, although Dr. M could imagine the patient breaking objects in the office, she did not consider herself in personal danger. Second, she took an inventory of her office contents. The sinking feeling persisted. Third, Dr. M attempted to determine how she would summon help if the situation got out of hand. Finally, she was aware of her intense anger and frustration. She felt that her next words needed to be carefully measured.

Dr. M [speaking with a cool, angry edge]: You could do that. It would certainly show me something. But I'd have to guess about what you were trying to show me. If you use words, it will communicate more clearly. Then, what is going on in you can be expressed and understood.

Ms. N: Oh, what do you know!? You think you are so in control. You have not helped me one bit. This sucks! When I leave here I'm going to kill myself. Why shouldn't I? What have you ever done for me? Did my mother ever want me? I have a way, you know. I know how to do it. But I won't tell you or anyone else about that.

Each of Ms. N's statements put another knot in the therapist's gut. At this point Dr. M was convinced that the patient was quite capable of doing as she threatened. Feeling painfully impotent and extremely angry, Dr. M suddenly wished the 7 minutes left in the hour were much longer. The thought of letting Ms. N walk out the door without some resolution was tormenting. The mounting anxiety, fear, and anger that Dr. M experienced at this moment was in sharp contrast to the absence of feeling in the first half of the session. Observing this dramatic shift in countertransference feelings, Dr. M attempted to analyze her own participation in a projective identification process. Concluding that the intensity of the countertransference was, in part, a communication from the patient, Dr. M responded.

Dr. M: Now I feel like hell. I'm concerned. I think you're making me feel the hell in you.
Ms. N [after a silence]: Now I feel sad.

Ms. N began to shed genuinely sad tears. She appeared three-dimensional for the first time in the therapy. Although Ms. N frequently cried, Dr. M had experienced the tears previously as an assault. This instance was decidedly different. The negative intensity of the countertransference reaction dissipated quickly. The therapist no longer saw the patient as an adversary. Rather, Ms. N seemed to be a vulnerable, sad, and frightened little girl.

Dr. M: I think it's nice that you can feel sad. Even though it's a tough feeling, I think it's very nice. [The patient continued to weep softly.] I shared the impact that you had on me. Now you're telling me about the impact on you. That's a genuine exchange. [As the hour drew to a close, Ms. N quietly walked out of the room.]

In the foregoing vignette, Dr. M made a carefully considered decision to disclose her own feelings to her patient. In so doing, she assisted Ms. N in making a shift from the paranoid-schizoid mode, in which she experienced her therapist as a persecutor driving her to suicide, to a depressive mode, in which she experienced genuine concern that her words and actions might have hurt her therapist. Her affect modulation greatly improved, and she was able to leave the session with her impulses under control.

A therapist's decision to engage in self-disclosure in a psychotherapy session with a borderline patient is fraught with difficulties. For example, in the case of Dr. M, she was aware that in certain moments her frustration with Ms. N had roots deep within her that were largely independent of the patient. Had she ventilated the frustration at such moments, she might have been at risk of using the patient for her own needs. However, Dr. M was well aware that certain other aspects of her emotional reaction to the patient were a joint creation of the patient's provocative behavior and the therapist's reaction to that behavior. When she recognized that the projective identification process was serving as a means of creating empathy in herself for what Ms. N was experiencing, she chose to share that impact with the patient.

The self-disclosure that we are suggesting as having circumscribed usefulness is not without its risks. Clinical honesty in the here-and-now must be carefully weighed in terms of its probable impact on a series of issues.

The Effect on
Transference Exploration

To get to the most primitive transference issues with borderline patients, therapists often have to waver on the brink of despair, at the point where their ability to continue effectively comes painfully into question (Gabbard 1991). Clearly, Dr. M reached this point in the therapy and decided to share it with Ms. N. Was Ms. N's subsequent ability to examine her own transference facilitated? Was it restricted?

Burke and Tansey (1991) observed that discussion of self-disclosure technique must be framed within a particular model of development and therapeutic action. For example, therapists adhering to a drive-conflict model of therapeutic action would argue that self-disclosure short-circuits the patient's regression to and development of a transference neurosis (Burke and Tansey 1991). As a result, whole arenas needing therapeutic examination are foreclosed. The minimal degree of countertransference self-disclosure advocated grows out of a technique designed for the expressive treatment of neurotic individuals. Borderline patients, in contrast, often require interventions that are much closer to the supportive end of the continuum. The ego weaknesses inherent in these individuals demand that the therapist be more active. From our point of view, the usefulness of countertransference self-disclosure must be reevaluated in this light.

The developmental-arrest model of therapeutic action directly addresses the patient's desperate and continuous search for someone who can be depended on for support (Burke and Tansey 1991). Empathic attunement is designed to help the patient move beyond past traumas that stunted self-development (Stolorow et al. 1987). Although countertransference reactions are viewed as important sources of information, self-disclosure by the therapist is considered an impingement of the therapist's self-experience on the patient's unfolding selfhood. The support offered is the therapist's responsibility to monitor and to sustain. The patient is seen as in no way contributing consciously, or unconsciously, to the therapist's countertransference dilemma and is understood as wishing for it to be otherwise (Burke and Tansey 1991).

Interpersonalists vary in their view of the value of self-disclosure depending on how they regard the therapeutic relationship along the axis of asymmetry versus mutuality (Burke 1992). Gill (1983), who articulated his concerns from the asymmetry perspective, suggested that too much self-disclosure shuts down exploration of the patient's subjective experience. Levenson (1983, 1990), on the other hand, stressed the mutuality in the psychotherapeutic situation, and he has argued that therapists must help patients understand how it feels to be involved with them in the interest of helping them get a clearer picture of both their own internal worlds and the impact they have on others.

In our view, the joint creation of the transference-countertransference paradigm cannot be underestimated. Ms. N presented with a dramatic, pseudoemotionality. She insisted that she felt nothing about Dr. M. Similarly, although notes written after the session suggested the opposite, Dr. M felt nothing in response. The very intense feelings toward each other, which both unconsciously harbored, were revealed finally through Dr. M's self-disclosure. Only after she became aware of the "hell" gripping her through the process of projective identification could Dr. M use words to present that experience for mutual consideration. At that point, and not before, Ms. N expressed genuine feelings for the first time in the course of the therapy. Dr. M's self-disclosure functioned as an infusion that dramatically transformed Ms. N's ability to reflect on her transference. Her complaints about the failings of the external world were replaced with an opportunity to sample, in a hateful manner, her sadness, concern, loneliness, guilt, and ambivalence. Ms. N's response also supports Burke's (1992) view that hearing about the therapist's feelings may actually diminish the patient's level of affective intensity.

Dr. M's ability to acknowledge, first to herself and then to the patient, that she felt more than "nothing" developed gradually over the sessions. She was increasingly able to tolerate the rage and helplessness that Ms. N was working so hard to induce in her. Carpy (1989) pointed out that the mutative aspects of tolerating the countertransference are distinct from the therapist's ability to remain unaffected by the patient's projections or to hide emotional responses from the patient. Tolerance of intense countertransference reflects the therapist's ability to permit the patient's projections to be experienced in their full force without acting on them in a gross way. If the projections are fully experienced, then the countertransference will inevitably be acted out to some partial degree (Carpy 1989).

Dr. M's coolly expressed anger at Ms. N's threat to destroy her office was apparent. Although Ms. N proceeded to batter Dr. M with complaints, her "actions" remained at the level of attacking words and did not spill over into attacking behavior. Presumably, by showing Ms. N her anger and implicitly holding her accountable, Dr. M introduced the opportunity for Ms. N to choose how she wanted to define herself (Ehrenberg 1984). Her own ego boundaries and the distinct existence of the therapist came more sharply into focus for her (Epstein 1977; Winnicott 1949). Dr. M's partial acting out enabled Ms. N to see, whether consciously or unconsciously, that she was affecting Dr. M by inducing strong feelings in her. The hell that Ms. N carried in her was identified through Dr. M's self-disclosure for their mutual consideration.

When Dr. M identified the "hell" that she felt within herself and then disclosed that experience to the patient, both felt relieved. By sharing her torturous impotence and rage, Dr. M identified the jointly created transference-countertransference paradigm and modified it by giving a bit of Ms. N's self back to her. Concurrently, Dr. M reclaimed her self as distinct from the patient and as a skilled clinician. This self-disclosure was useful to them both, because both were extricated from the transference-countertransference enactment in a fashion that allowed reflection on the mutual exchange between them.

Although self-disclosure may provide relief from countertransference discomfort, the goal should never be for the singular purpose of easing the therapist's experience. Bollas (1983) elegantly stated that no therapist "should only interpret to relieve himself of the psychic pain he may be in, but equally, neither should he be ignorant of those interpretations that cure him of the patient's effect" (p. 14).

The Impact on Neutrality

Is therapeutic neutrality lost if the therapist is something other than anonymous and abstinent with the patient? Historically, neutrality was first defined by Anna Freud (1936/1966), who said that the analyst "takes his stand at a point equidistant from the id, the ego, and the superego" (p. 28). Since that time, the concept has unfortunately been misused to connote *detachment* from the patient instead of the original meaning of a nonjudgmental posture. Greenberg (1986b) pointed out how maintaining the proper neutral "place" is nearly impossible to do. For example, developing a working alliance with the patient is a departure from neutrality, because it establishes a collaboration with one part of the psychic structure (the patient's observing ego) at the expense of the other systems.

Behaviors occurring in the name of neutrality are simply one way of participating in the therapeutic dialogue and are no less likely to influence that dialogue than any other way of participating (Greenberg 1986b; Wachtel 1982). To conceive of neutrality as embodied in a set of behaviors, Greenberg (1986a, 1986b) argued, is misplaced. Rather, neutrality should be considered the goal of the therapist's behavior. The patient's experience of safety, which is intimately connected to the perception of past traumas, betrayals, seductions, and the like, hangs in the balance between perceiving the therapist as the old, dangerous, and disappointed object, or as a new and different object.

As noted in Chapter 2, Greenberg (1986a, 1986b) defined the goal of neutrality as the therapist's striking a balance between being perceived as an old object and a new object. With this understanding, silence and anonymity enable patients to include the therapist in their internal object world, whereas more active interventions, including self-disclosure, establish the therapist as a new object. Accordingly, "neutrality . . . is not to be measured by the analyst's behaviors at any moment, but by the particular patient's ability to become aware of and to tolerate his transference" (Greenberg 1986a, p. 97).

In our view, focusing on neutrality as a goal and not as a set of behaviors has particular relevance for the treatment of borderline patients. Neutrality as a construct involving anonymity and equidistance is simply not tenable with these patients (Searles 1986). The need to work with these individuals in a manner that is both expressive and supportive calls for flexibility. More specifically, the loss of the "as if" nature of transference described in Chapter 2 leads these patients to be highly prone to approach *all* relationships as if the other person were simply an actor from their internal drama. For example, they are likely to insist that their therapist is the *same* punitive, disappointing maternal figure whom they have suffered in the past. Yet, simultaneously, such individuals will urgently implore the therapist to care for them in a fashion that they never experienced as a child. Greenberg (1986a) astutely observed that, "if the analyst cannot be experienced as a new object, analysis never gets underway; if he cannot be experienced as an old one, it never ends" (p. 98). Borderline patients both desperately need this balance and attempt to disrupt it at every turn.

For borderline patients constrained by the part-object relationships of their internal world, the therapist's self-disclosure can function as a means to achieve a neutral balance. For the self-revelation to be useful in establishing, consolidating, or restoring neutrality, therapists must assess the degree to which they have been cast into the role of the old or the new object. When the patient's attribution of one or the other is absolute, the neutral balance is lost. Moreover, in that moment, the patient's static inner experience is taken as a true representation of the external world. Therapists are simply who their patients perceive them to be. The unidimensionality of the patient's experience forecloses exploration. The task of establishing inner openness *and* learning how to inhabit it fall to the therapist (Lewin and Schulz 1992).

Awareness of countertransference reactions can prove invaluable at this juncture. Listening to the patient's attributions, while simultaneously attending to countertransference associations, assists the therapist in linking lost aspects of the patient's self with the use of the therapist. The complementarity between the patient's transference and the therapist's countertransference is reflected in the complementarity of the therapist's listening and talking, or self-disclosing. Both modes of experience and discourse inform and deepen the therapeutic process (Lewin and Schulz 1992).

Countertransference reflection provides a therapeutic lens through which therapists can observe how their patients are using them as objects (Bollas 1983). "Objectification" of one's personal experience allows the therapist to determine what interventions would restore a neutral state. For example, Ms. N complained repeatedly about helpers letting her down. Dr. M first listened, then asked for elaboration. Yet, thoughtful listening, empathy, and attempted transference interpretations did not deepen an understanding of Ms. N's complaints, which simply grew more emphatic. Dr. M felt increasingly helpless and annoyed. A dangerous loss of neutrality threatened as the transference-countertransference paradigm became more and more constrained. The opportunity existed for Dr. M to become like the old, frustrating, rejecting maternal object. By actively waving her hands to interrupt Ms. N's increasingly action-oriented behavior, and ultimately disclosing that she, too, felt like hell, Dr. M established herself as a new and distinct object. A balance between the old dangers and the new possibilities was established.

The Influence on Patient Revelations

The type of information revealed by the patient subsequent to the therapist's self-disclosure is influenced by that disclosure. The same can be said, however, of the type of information that the patient reveals subsequent to the therapist's silence. From our point of view, the therapist must track the patient's associations, whether in response to abstinence or self-disclosure. The emphasis is on understanding the joint transference-countertransference creation that is unfolding, rather than attempting to influence it.

When a self-disclosure has been offered to the patient, watching for the reactions, both conscious and unconscious, is imperative. Without an awareness of the patient's response, therapists are in danger of falling prey to their own need to be right (Hoffman 1983). As a result, countertransference inordinately influences the therapeutic process through the therapist's dependence on subjective experience and the patient's resisted ideas about the therapist's subjective experience. Despite the patient's resistances to acknowledging perceptions of the countertransference, the therapist must ultimately clarify and work through the interaction. To do otherwise leaves a transference-countertransference enactment unattended.

Returning to the work with Ms. N, we can see the facilitating effects of Dr. M's disclosures. However, the positive transference that developed spawned intense envy that had to be addressed, as illustrated in a later session.

Ms. N began the hour by uncharacteristically volunteering that she valued the therapy. She reflected on her sense of inner "emptiness" and then recalled that she had often pretended to be the story character Heidi as a child. It was the first reference in the course of the treatment to warm, personally meaningful childhood fantasies.

Heidi's story also had been a favorite of Dr. M's as a child. The warmth of the moment felt too good to pass up, and Dr. M recounted several scenes to their mutual pleasure. At the end of the hour, Ms. N expressed her appreciation at being able to share memories of the story with Dr. M.

In the next session, after describing in great detail other fantasy relationships, Ms. N paused to say that she felt "silly" about having such daydreams. Dr. M's query led to the patient's recollection that her mother had often intruded on her fantasy play. To this day, she felt like she had to protect carefully her imaginary playmates from someone else's harsh criticism. Dr. M gently pointed out that Ms. N's "companions," as well as the richness of her fantasies, was evidence that she was not "empty." Ms. N appeared grateful that her treasured friends and their adventures had been respected.

The following day Ms. N ragefully asserted that she destroyed everything good that she built. As proof she angrily described how she stamped out every anthill that she could find as a child. She called herself evil and despicable for ruining the home of innocent ants. Dr. M's thoughts wandered to an ant farm that she had had as a child. She recalled watching with fascination as the ants burrowed between the plates of glass to construct an elaborate underground home. She also recalled that on more than one occasion she had inserted her finger through the feeding hole at the top and smoothed over the entrances to the burrows. Again with fascination, she watched as the ants efficiently rebuilt their damaged thresholds.

The metaphor of object constancy embodied in her associations to the ant farm flashed through Dr. M's mind. The ability of the ants to rebuild seemed to be a continuation on the theme of recent sessions that building a helpful relationship was possible despite shifting thoughts, feelings, and behaviors. In contrast to the devastation the patient attributed to her stomping on the anthill entrances, the resiliency of the ants the therapist remembered suggested that what happens underneath is not always consistent with surface appearances.

Dr. M decided to describe in detail her childhood experience of that ant farm. Ms. N appeared enchanted—less by the content of the story than the discovery that Dr. M could weave together her personal memories. As the session closed, Ms. N said, "I really appreciate your telling me about the ant farm. I never would have guessed that you had one."

Ms. N began the subsequent session by stormily berating herself for "undermining" the treatment through her ever-present "envy." She reasoned that Dr. M had quite artfully offered her an opportunity for growth and that she had destroyed that chance. Dr. M recognized a countertransference pull to agree with Ms. N's assertion that her envy was a countertherapeutic force. However, Dr. M, silently analyzing the progression of the hour, inferred that Ms. N's envy stemmed from her unrealistic perception that her profound dependency needs could only be met through the therapist's benevolent attention. Consequently, for Dr. M to affirm Ms. N's envy would tacitly reinforce a pathological self- and object-representation in which Ms. N was profoundly inadequate and Dr. M alone held all the power to meet her needs. If such a scenario were true, then a burning sense of envy would be appropriate.

Dr. M decided to intervene by strongly asserting that the good work occurring in the therapy was not due to the therapist's outstanding skills alone. Rather, the good work could only be understood as a collaborative effort. The patient's contribution was just as essential as that of the therapist's, and the success of the therapy depended on what they could do together.

In the following meeting Ms. N asked Dr. M to help her address a serious problem that Ms. N had previously minimized. Dr. M silently noted that Ms. N appeared to be making a nascent effort to draw on both internal and external resources rather than reflexively acting out.

Spontaneous self-disclosure, such as Dr. M's enthusiastic discussion about Heidi, always risks being an enactment of a countertransferential blind spot. As a result, the patient's subsequent revelations may be profoundly affected by the shifting focus from the patient's use of the therapist to the therapist's use of the patient. Dr. M, although entirely spontaneous in her remarks, did not transgress this boundary. She did not use Ms. N to gratify her personal needs. Rather, Dr. M's acknowledgment of mutual interests appeared to facilitate further revelations by the patient.

Masterson (1976) advocated similar forms of discussion with patients, using Mahler's (Mahler et al. 1975) notion of communicative matching as a conceptual framework. In this context, Masterson acknowledged that sharing knowledge about mutual areas of interest (e.g., current events, film, sports) may provide the patient with an experience of validation from caretakers that was lacking during childhood development, thus moving the patient toward autonomy and individuation. He suggested that this limited form of self-disclosure is most helpful when a newly emerging aspect of the patient's self becomes apparent. However, he stressed that such discussions must stem from a sense of attunement to the patient and not the narcissistic needs of the therapist. Obviously, such discussions entail a partial transference gratification for the patient, and the extent to which the therapy is conceptualized as supportive rather than expressive will be an important determinant of how often the therapist indulges in such discussions with the patient.

Despite the usefulness of acknowledging shared interests, the therapist must assess the degree to which self-disclosure embodies a personal blind spot. All therapists who pursue intensive therapeutic work with borderline patients should have their own treatment experience. Subsequent to terminating, therapists should pursue rigorous self-analysis, and if necessary, consultation. However, as

Sandler (1976) noted:

> Very often the irrational response of the (therapist), which his pro-
> fessional conscience leads him to see entirely as a blind spot of his
> own, may sometimes be usefully regarded as a compromise-forma-
> tion between his own tendencies and *his reflexive acceptance of the role*
> *which the patient is forcing on him.* (p. 46)

Dr. M's description of her own ant farm was particularly uncharacteristic of her technique. In retrospect, Dr. M realized that
Ms. N wished and feared that her past experience with an intrusive,
controlling, and omnipotent mother would be repeated. If that specific relational paradigm had been enacted, Ms. N would have been
on familiar ground, and she could have continued to rail against
her victimization. Dr. M unconsciously sidestepped the maternal
projection and, instead, identified with the child. As two little girls,
they discussed a shared experience. Thus the compromise formation, which Sandler (1976) described, allowed Dr. M to lend her
ego resources to Ms. N as a peer rather than as a hated authority
figure.

Presumably, Dr. M's independence from the object of projection was initially reassuring to Ms. N, and subsequently disquieting.
Through making Ms. N's envious reactions to Dr. M's disclosure explicit and clarifying their mutual contribution, Ms. N was ultimately
able to ask in a collaborative manner for assistance on a previously
denied problem.

Do self-disclosures by therapists help patients discover more
about themselves? Or, are patients less likely to reveal information?
From our point of view, the interpersonal and intrapsychic nuances
developing both within and between the patient and the therapist,
if brought into awareness, can convey far more about the patient's
inner world than words alone. Racker's (1957) seminal article on
the concordant and complementary identifications inherent in
countertransference paved the way for many others to explore how
the patient's internal object world can be discovered through the
therapist's personal reactions (Ogden 1982; Scharff 1992; Stolorow
et al. 1983).

Once therapists have discovered fragments of the patient's internal object world within their personal experience, they are in a better position to help the patient distinguish between old, subjectively dangerous, internally derived objects and new, potentially mutative, external objects. For example, Dr. M was initially unaware of having introjected an aspect of Ms. N. Consciously, Dr. M felt nothing, although the parapraxis evidenced in her notes suggested that her bland reaction was a defensive maneuver to keep "*me* from telling *you* about *my pain.*" Through ongoing interactions with Ms. N, Dr. M eventually discovered that pain and described it like the "hell" that it was. As a result, Ms. N shifted from a unidimensional self-experience to a newer, fuller sense of self that included guilt, empathy, warmth, and depressive anxieties.

Borderline patients, almost by definition, preemptively dismiss large chunks of their personal experience. Self-disclosure, such as Dr. M's recognition of "feeling like hell," can help patients make links in their internal world that they had been unable to do for themselves. Bollas (1983) pointed out that to the degree the patient makes himself or herself known through the therapist's experience, the other source of the patient's free associations is the therapist's countertransference—so much so that at times the therapist's free associations may be the only associations informing the process. The following vignette illustrates how the patient needed the therapist to have real feelings before she could permit human reactions in herself.

After waiting for quite some time, Mrs. M and her husband had adopted a little girl. Within 2 years of entering the family, it became evident that the child, Tricia, had to be placed in a therapeutic nursery for autistic and developmentally disabled children. The child had also developed a seizure disorder that had required a long and arduous treatment course with many setbacks. Mrs. M had entered therapy when Tricia was 8 years old, seeking help for her own depressive reaction.

Two years into therapy, Mrs. M began the session by presenting her therapist, Dr. N, with two cartoons. One pictured a patient driving a bulldozer toward a psychotherapist while commenting she had no particular associations to his question. The second depicted a patient making a crass statement about the psychotherapist's latent hostility. When asked if she was trying to communicate something about anger, Mrs. M patronizingly suggested that Dr. N took his job too seriously. She went on to describe dispassionately her daughter's most recent seizure episode.

The matter-of-fact manner in which Mrs. M described the latest downturn of her daughter's course was disquieting to Dr. N. The family had suffered one tragedy after another, although no one could not gauge their travails by the patient's affectless account. Based on past experience, Dr. N knew that this manner of speaking about extremely troubling experiences was quite expectable for this woman. It was not so much a depressive mask as a primary aspect of her character structure. Although Mrs. M and Dr. N had arrived at many insights over the course of the therapy regarding the interrelationship between her childhood experiences in an alcoholic home and her current situation, Mrs. M could not rid herself of a nagging sense of alienation and ineptness in her relationship to others. Typically, she covered over her perplexity by convincing herself that she was an extraordinary crisis manager.

Mrs. M continued by explaining that her daughter had to be hospitalized because of the neurologist's grave concern. She then reported that Tricia's orthopedist felt that the window of opportunity for some long-delayed corrective surgery would be soon closed. Also, since the last session, Mrs. M had spoken to Tricia's psychotherapist, who had suggested that the first incidence of the child's psychogenic headaches had been at the time of Mr. M's mother's death. Mrs. M recounted blandly and in great detail how her mother-in-law, to whom Tricia had been quite close, died suddenly of kidney failure 6 years earlier. Dr. N imagined that the events around the death must have been very painful for the whole family, confusing for a little girl, and perplexing to the parents of a 4-year-old.

Brimming with reactions, Dr. N found Mrs. M's understated, emotionless presentation incredulous. As the patient continued to speak, Dr. N became more and more concerned about Tricia's medical and psychiatric treatment. He began to fantasize about making arrangements for the child to be admitted to a hospital unit specializing in the psychiatric evaluation of physically ill children.

Spurred on by Mrs. M's complacency, Dr. N disclosed his growing sense of concern *and* urgency regarding the daughter's treatment needs. He had made such comments many times before in an effort to communicate to Mrs. M that feelings were a natural and enriching aspect of human relating and not a sign of terminal vulnerability. When Mrs. M responded that the treatment course would be a long one and that "urgency" was not a factor, Dr. N observed that urgency could also be associated with a sense of impending crisis. He was well aware that Mrs. M had stirred a sense of crisis in him.

At this moment, Mrs. M's depersonalized reckoning began to take on a more human quality. In an abstract fashion she described her worries about her child and her doubts about her adequacy as a parent. While Dr. N continued to speak about the affect stirred in him by the gulf between Mrs. M's woeful family situation and her feelings, the patient's cognitive appraisal of the situation began to diminish. Some of the perplexity dominating her inner world began to show through.

Mrs. M's casual rehash of events and reactions belied her caricatured adaptation to the passionate aspects of human loving, hurting, losing, hating, and grieving. Her transference of detachment had been understood. Mrs. M could easily cite numerous insights regarding her memories as a helpless child in the shadow of a selfish, drunken mother. Yet insights alone had not been able to unlock her emotional prison (S. Freud 1916–1917/1961). By reifying her affects, Mrs. M unconsciously hoped to change her painful reality. The result, instead, was to make herself into an automaton. Dr. N's affective contribution was crucial in helping Mrs. M acknowledge her alienation, fear of ineptitude, and perplexity (Ehrenberg 1984).

Rosenfeld (1971) distinguished between the patient's use of projective identification as a *communication* and its use as a *disavowal of psychic reality*. In the former, the patient is much more likely to receive the therapist's interpretation as personally meaningful. In the latter, the same interpretation may be experienced as a forced reentry (Carpy 1989). An analogy to this distinction can be applied to the return of the projected contents from the therapist back to the patient. Dr. N could not shove the grave concern he encountered regarding Tricia's condition back at Mrs. M when she did not consciously feel any concern. To have done so would have confirmed for her that such distressing reactions are intolerable and must be eliminated through projective evacuation. However, over the course of the session, Dr. N's increasingly obvious concern allowed Mrs. M to see, consciously or unconsciously, that her situation induced strong feelings that could be managed. Through this very gradual process, Mrs. M had begun to discover aspects of herself in Dr. N's reactions.

The task before Mrs. M and Dr. N extended beyond the reclamation of her affective experience. Her ability to experience her "self-with-other" was fundamentally disrupted (Stern 1983). Dr. N's tolerance of the intolerable aspects of the patient's self, together with his display of the distress that she induced, allowed her the positive, contact-making opportunity inherent in the projective process (Lewin and Schulz 1992). Although in a small increment, Mrs. M relinquished her detachment and availed herself to a new category of experience that "can never even occur unless elicited or maintained by the actions of another and would never exist as a part of known self-experience without another" (Stern 1983, p. 74).

Direct Versus Indirect Self-Disclosure

Dr. N acknowledged his concern about Mrs. M's daughter through reference to feelings that Mrs. M had not yet articulated about herself. Bollas (1983) suggested that we label as indirect uses of countertransference interventions organized around what the therapist senses about the patient's self. Accordingly, the goal of indirect use of countertransference is to enable the patient increasingly to trust the value of expressing as yet unknowable subjective states. Bollas differentiated this therapeutic task from the much rarer direct use of countertransference when therapists describe their experience as the patient's object. Although we agree with Bollas that the direct use of countertransference must be used judiciously, we would add that we are more likely to speak directly about the patient's use of the therapist as an object with borderline patients than with higher-functioning individuals. Simply put, borderline patients need more help distinguishing between their internal objects that have been projected onto the external world and the actual external world.

The degree of directness is determined by the patient's capacity to contain an affective experience of self in relation to other. The therapist should not use self-disclosure if to do so pushes patients beyond their capacity for containment. As Lewin and Schulz (1992) pointed out, what is crucial is "not what we can do *for* the patient, but what we can do *with* the patient" (p. 316). In the following vignette, the therapist could do little *for* the patient to help effect change. However, in being *with* the patient in a fresh way, change occurred.

Several years into the treatment process, when rehashing a familiar and previously unproductive topic, Mrs. L uncharacteristically became receptive to interpretations about how she repeatedly pushed Ms. O, a clinical social worker, away. As a result, she described new genetic material in which revealing an aspect of herself to others meant a loss of her autonomy.

Mrs. L began the next session by saying that she had felt understood by Ms. O for the first time. Next, she announced that she was seeking consultation with her marital therapist about the possibility of beginning individual therapy with him. Ms. O inquired what Mrs. L hoped the marital therapist could provide that the patient found lacking in the current psychotherapy process. Vaguely, Mrs. L explained that the marital therapist knew her family better and that she had the luxury of not having to explain about the important people in her life. Besides, she recalled conversations in which Ms. O had pointed out to her that maybe she did not want to change if it meant painfully turning her insides out.

As Mrs. L proceeded with the marital therapy consultation and made plans to terminate with Ms. O, her behavior became quite ambiguous. She spoke of getting nowhere with Ms. O, of extreme dissatisfaction, but chose a termination date that was 5 months away. Ms. O was quite confused about whether to confront her flight from being "understood for the first time," or to support her adaptive retreat in the face of being turned painfully inside out. Both confrontational and supportive interventions yielded ambiguous results. For example, Mrs. L acted within the sessions as if she intended to stay there forever. Yet, when this style of interacting was pointed out to her, she firmly held to her intentions to leave several months hence. Based on a diagnostic understanding that the only conditions under which this woman could become closer was to know that she always had the option to leave, Ms. O decided not to speak directly about termination with her.

In the course of their discussions, Mrs. L woefully observed that she wanted to stay "secretive, powerful, and in control" by operating with absolute independence. But at the same time, Mrs. L longed to feel understood and close. She sadly noted that if she moved toward allowing others to understand her, she would feel inside out. If she moved toward absolute independence, she would feel cut off. Even though the dilemma surrounding her termination plans had been mutually acknowledged, Ms. O still had no idea what Mrs. L intended to do.

One month after feeling exceptionally well understood, Mrs. L admonished Ms. O not to "come after" her and drag her back into the psychotherapy process. She related how people had taken such actions against her all of her life. For example, her mother had not wanted her to leave home, or to get married, or to have children, or to get an education. Her mother had just wanted the patient to stay and take care of her. This time she simply was not going to stand for it.

The more Mrs. L warned Ms. O not to chase after her, the more the therapist felt an intense desire to do so. In fact, the image flashed through the therapist's mind that Mrs. L would jump out of her chair in the next instant and head for the door. In that moment, Ms. O literally sat on her hands and figuratively bit her tongue to keep herself from saying anything to the patient that would seem to be an effort to influence Mrs. L to stay. Strangely, when that session ended, Ms. O still did not know whether Mrs. L planned to terminate or not.

By gradually disclosing in the next few sessions her own anxiety regarding Mrs. L's leaving, Ms. O helped Mrs. L acknowledge the anxiety as her own. Mrs. L spoke for the first time about her concern that she was doing the wrong thing. Moreover, Mrs. L revealed that she believed that no therapy or therapist could ever ease her situation because she was incapable of changing. She intended to remain miserable rather than face the profound grief and uncertainty that existed deeper in her experience. She had no plans for what she wanted to work on with her next therapist and was not interested in formulating any. She would just go and talk to him.

In her last hour, Mrs. L spoke for the first time about her previous two therapists. She observed that she had left the first one behind without any warning. The second one she had met with once to say goodbye. Her extended termination process with Ms. O was quite unusual by contrast. Ms. O pointed out that she had opened up a bit more with each succeeding therapist. Maybe she could only go so far with one before she had to move on to the next one. Mrs. L nodded her head affirmatively as she minimized the significance of the current therapy. She was quite surprised when Ms. O said that she would be pleased to hear from the patient in the future.

Ms. O had very few options initially for helping Mrs. L reflect on her flight. Even the most benign, indirect use of countertransference to illuminate Mrs. L's self-experience would have pushed her far beyond her capacity for containment. As a result, the uncertain situation would have been prematurely forced into an enactment of an internal object relationship that was entirely unconscious, introducing a new, less dangerous object to the situation.

What facilitated Ms. O's eventual indirect use of countertransference was Mrs. L's correct identification of Ms. O's wish to "come after" her. Interpersonalists such as Hoffman (1983), Aron (1991), and Mitchell (1988) have invited us to consider the patient's perception of the therapist's subjectivity as part of the transference. Mrs. L knew at some level that she was influencing Ms. O's experience and that Ms. O had only limited freedom to resist that influence. By recognizing Mrs. L's interpretation as an indication of Mrs. L's transference *and* being conscious of her own side of the repetition in the countertransference, Ms. O was able to shed light on Mrs. L's painful compromise. Although Ms. O did little *for* Mrs. L, being *with* her in a different way changed her manner of saying goodbye.

The Link Between
Understanding and Self-Disclosure

As we stressed in Chapter 2, the most ordinary state of countertransference involves experiencing without yet knowing (Bollas 1983). Understanding the borderline patient's use of the object and sense of self very often requires observation of how the therapist is being used. If therapists can abide by a loss of their personal sense of identity in this clinical crucible, they are better able to achieve the necessary "process identity" that allows for reception and registration of the patient's transference (Bollas 1983). Hirsch (1987) aptly noted that the observing part of the therapist often does not help avoid becoming involved in some form of transference-countertransference enactment. However, the therapist's observing, analytic ego does allow the enactment to be seen once it is in process. The therapeutic task is to examine the process identity evoked in the therapist and to clarify what the engagement between the patient and therapist has become. Then the effort of working through can begin (Bollas 1983; Hirsch 1987).

Dr. M did not fully understand the hellish experience that she shared with Ms. N. Similarly, Dr. N could not predict with certainty how Mrs. M would make use of the "real" feelings evoked by her tragic circumstances. Ms. O did not know whether or not she should dare to acknowledge the pressure and confusion within herself. If any of these therapists had spoken to their subjective experience as if it were the official psychoanalytic decoding of the patient's inner world, the result would have been a potentially harmful display of arrogance. The challenge before each was to make known to the patient a private, subjective experience that might inform their mutual analytic investigation. Bollas (1983), paying tribute to Winnicott, suggested that the therapist needs to play with the patient by offering countertransference disclosures as if they were objects that are meant to be passed back and forth between the two. Here the therapist's attitude is equally as important as the content of the disclosure. If therapists can relate their own subjective experiences as objects to be kicked around, mulled over, torn to pieces, thereby offering the opportunity to release the patient toward a new self-experience, then absolute understanding of the countertransference is not a prerequisite for its use as a therapeutic tool (Bollas 1983).

The risk in self-disclosing feelings before they are fully understood is that the patient may feel burdened to provide meaning to the therapist's emotional state (Burke 1992; Hoffman 1983). Although some patients may benefit from this experience, others may be overwhelmed by it. Based on this concern, many therapists attempt to formulate meaning as part of the self-disclosure.

Nonverbal Self-Disclosure

The focus of this chapter on the delineation of the circumstances in which a therapist should verbalize countertransference feelings to a patient runs the risk of minimizing the role of ongoing self-disclosure that occurs at a nonverbal level. Rayner (1992) drew on the infant observations of Stern (1985) to apply the analogy of the affective attunement that occurs between mother and infant. He observed that a good deal of "acting" or "playing" goes on between analyst and patient in the same way that it does between mother and child, a process that constitutes an affective "duet." Although Rayner acknowledged the differences between an adult patient in analysis and the mother-child setting, he suggested that such attunement approximates preverbal rhythms occurring developmentally and therefore may precede verbal interpretations. Whether the treatment is conducted vis-à-vis or using the couch, therapists respond in a way that partially imitates the patient's mood and communicates to the patient that the affect has been received and is being shared. Rayner (1992) noted: "Words may alienate or falsify. With this in mind, I have suggested that vocal, but pre-verbal, affect-attunement exchanges may be a necessary precursor to meaningful verbal exchanges in analysis" (p. 49).

Rayner (1992) made the point that therapists are communicating a good deal about their internal states without ever directly expressing countertransference feelings to the patient. The mothers that Stern (1985) observed were not unnecessarily burdening their children with emotional outbursts. Rayner, commenting on Stern's research, noted:

> They were focusing deeply upon their child's activity and affect, then reacting with attuned affect to him. Their feelings seem to have been free moving yet coherent. In classical terms, the feelings were sublimated ones. This is what the analyst in touch with his patient does, at least quietly to himself. (p. 52)

The point we wish to stress here is that communications about the therapist's internal state are continually being conveyed to the patient through vocalizations, facial expressions, tone of voice, and physical activity. The therapist's feelings emerge in small doses throughout the course of treatment. Aron (1991) noted that "self-revelation is not an option; it is an inevitability" (p. 40).

Responses to Direct Questions

The foregoing discussion of the indirect expression of the therapist's feelings is closely linked to the so-called radar that many observers have attributed to borderline patients. Rather than invoking the presence of telepathic powers, we would submit that this phenomenon of being sensitive to the therapist's feelings is a direct result of the borderline patient's tendency to evoke strong affective states in the therapist that are difficult to disguise. The radar is simply a way of describing the patient's observations of a plethora of nonverbal communications of the therapist's emotional states.

A predictable result of the patient's observation of the therapist is for the patient to make direct inquiries regarding the therapist's feelings. All therapists of borderline patients will be asked sooner or later such questions as, "Are you angry at me?" "Do you hate me?" and "Am I boring you?" Therapists must carefully choose their answers to such questions because the patient is potentially vulnerable to serious narcissistic injury. An errant or impulsive answer may even lead to a disruption of the treatment.

Questions about the therapist's feelings must first be considered in the same light as all questions. Is it best to give a direct answer or to explore the patient's thoughts about the question? Often the response to a question will be determined by the degree to which the psychotherapy is conceptualized as expressive versus supportive. In other words, the more supportive the therapy, the more likely the therapist is to provide direct answers to questions. Another option favored by some interpersonalists is to describe one's response to being asked the question (Burke 1992).

In attempting to offer guidelines for the therapist, we return to the concept of clinical honesty mentioned earlier in the chapter. One time-honored rule of thumb in the treatment of borderline patients is to avoid dishonesty. If the therapist is angry at the patient but denies it, such a response compounds the difficulty. In addition to the knowledge that the therapist is angry, the patient also knows that the therapist is dishonest. The patient will then wonder, "If the therapist lies in this situation, am I also being lied to in other situations?"

Having established that honesty is essential in formulating responses to such questions, the next issue that bears on the therapist's answer is tact. Telling a patient "I hate you" is rarely helpful. When possible, therapists should try to couch their responses in terms that suggest that an interaction is taking place that has produced the emotional state in the therapist. Instead of saying, "I hate you," a therapist might reply, "I think you are correct that I am starting to feel angry, and I think it would be useful for us to explore together how I've come to feel this way." The therapist can then explore what behaviors or comments from the patient have produced feelings of anger and how they might be repeating a pattern that has occurred in other relationships.

Certainly there are some statements a therapist must never make to the patient. In addition to "I hate you," it is never productive for a therapist to say "You bore me," because the therapist has not contracted for entertainment when a psychotherapy process has begun. Casement (1985) described a tactful way of dealing with countertransference boredom. He examined with the patient the way she is relating to him and said, "I have noticed, for some time now, that you frequently speak to me as if you are not expecting me to be interested in what you are saying" (p. 68). In this manner, he sensitively brought up his own responses without hurting the patient's feelings and with the suggestion that the patient's manner of relating is directly linked to his response to her.

Summary

In summarizing our suggestions regarding self-disclosure, we would like to emphasize Harry Stack Sullivan's (1954) observation that the uniqueness of psychotherapy lies in the fact that therapists put aside their own needs in the interest of addressing the patient's needs. Unloading our feelings on the patient simply because those feelings are difficult to bear is certainly an abuse of psychotherapy. However, as noted in Chapter 5, all therapists will reach a point when they simply cannot go on in a therapeutically effective way if they do not make some effort to reflect back the nature of the impact the patient is having on them. Direct sharing of this sort may help identify jointly created transference-countertransference enactments that are therapeutically useful.

Although self-disclosures may have an effect on the patient's subsequent associations and revelations, failure to disclose powerful affects will also influence the patient. No simple guidelines can be provided. As Burke (1992) noted: "Rules of thumb tend to diminish one's receptivity to the subtleties of the interaction and produce a locked-in or autopilot feel to the therapist's responsiveness" (p. 268). In a sensitive psychotherapy process, self-disclosure is occurring continually. The real issues for the therapist are to what extent feelings should be articulated and what mode of communication will maximize tact and minimize hurt.

References

Aron L: The patient's experience of the analyst's subjectivity. Psychoanalytic Dialogues 1:29–51, 1991

Bollas C: Expressive uses of the countertransference: notes to the patient from oneself. Contemporary Psychoanalysis 19:1–34, 1983

Burke WF: Countertransference disclosure and the asymmetry/mutuality dilemma. Psychoanalytic Dialogues 2:241–271, 1992

Burke WF, Tansey MJ: Countertransference disclosure and models of therapeutic action. Contemporary Psychoanalysis 27:351–384, 1991

Carpy DV: Tolerating the countertransference: a mutative process. Int J Psychoanal 70:287–294, 1989

Casement P: Further Learning From the Patient. London, Tavistock, 1985

Ehrenberg DB: Psychoanalytic engagement, II: affective considerations. Contemporary Psychoanalysis 20:560–583, 1984

Epstein L: The therapeutic function of hate in the countertransference. Contemporary Psychoanalysis 13:442–468, 1977

Freud A: The Writings of Anna Freud, Volume 2: The Ego and the Mechanisms of Defense (1936), Revised Edition. Translated by Baines C. New York, International Universities Press, 1966

Freud S: Introductory lectures on psycho-analysis (1916–1917), in The Standard Edition of the Complete Psychological Works of Sigmund Freud, Vol 15–16. Translated and edited by Strachey J. London, Hogarth Press, 1961, pp 1–482

Gabbard GO: Technical approaches to transference hate in the analysis of borderline patients. Int J Psychoanal 72:625–637, 1991

Gill M: The interpersonal paradigm and the degree of the therapist's involvement. Contemporary Psychoanalysis 19:200–237, 1983

Greenberg JR: The problem of analytic neutrality. Contemporary Psychoanalysis 22:76–86, 1986a

Greenberg JR: Theoretical models and the analyst's neutrality. Contemporary Psychoanalysis 22:87–106, 1986b

Gutheil T, Gabbard GO: The concept of boundaries in clinical practice: theoretical and risk management dimensions. Am J Psychiatry 150:188–196, 1993

Hirsch I: Varying modes of analytic participation. J Am Acad Psychoanal 15:205–222, 1987

Hoffman IZ: The patient as interpreter of the analyst's experience. Contemporary Psychoanalysis 19:389–422, 1983

Levenson EA: The Ambiguity of Change: An Inquiry into the Nature of Psychoanalytic Reality. New York, Basic Books, 1983

Levenson EA: Reply to Hoffman. Contemporary Psychoanalysis 26:299–304, 1990

Lewin RA, Schulz CG: Losing and Fusing: Borderline and Transitional Object and Self Relations. Northvale, NJ, Jason Aronson, 1992

Mahler MS, Pine F, Bergman A: The Psychological Birth of the Human Infant: Symbiosis and Individuation. New York, Basic Books, 1975

Masterson JF: Psychotherapy of the Borderline Adult: A Developmental Approach. New York, Brunner/Mazel, 1976

Mitchell SA: Relational Concepts in Psychoanalysis: An Integration. Cambridge, MA, Harvard University Press, 1988

Ogden TH: Projective Identification and Psychotherapeutic Technique. New York, Jason Aronson, 1982

Racker H: The meanings and uses of countertransference. Psychoanal Q 26:303–357, 1957

Rayner E: Matching, attunement and the psychoanalytic dialogue. Int J Psychoanal 73:39–54, 1992

Rosenfeld HE: Contribution to the psychopathology of psychotic states: the importance of projective identification in the ego structure and the object relations of the psychotic patient, in Problems of Psychosis. Edited by Doucet P, Laurin C. Amsterdam, Excerpta Medica, 1971, pp 115–128

Sandler J: Countertransference and role-responsiveness. International Review of Psychoanalysis 3:43–47, 1976

Scharff JS: Projective and Introjective Identification and the Use of the Therapist's Self. Northvale, NJ, Jason Aronson, 1992

Searles HF: My Work With Borderline Patients. Northvale, NJ, Jason Aronson, 1986

Stern DN: The early development of schemas of self, other, and "self with other," in Reflections on Self Psychology. Edited by Lichtenberg JD, Kaplan S. Hillsdale, NJ, Analytic Press, 1983, pp 49–84

Stern DN: The Interpersonal World of the Infant: A View From Psychoanalysis and Developmental Psychology. New York, Basic Books, 1985

Stolorow RD, Brandchaft B, Atwood GE: Intersubjectivity in psychoanalytic treatment: with special reference to archaic states. Bull Menninger Clin 47:117–128, 1983

Stolorow RD, Brandchaft B, Atwood GE: Psychoanalytic Treatment: An Intersubjective Approach. Hillsdale, NJ, Analytic Press, 1987

Sullivan HS: The Psychiatric Interview. New York, WW Norton, 1954

Wachtel PL: Vicious circles: the self and the rhetoric of emerging and unfolding. Contemporary Psychoanalysis 18:259–273, 1982

Winnicott DW: Hate in the counter-transference. Int J Psychoanal 30:69–74, 1949

CHAPTER 8

Splitting

Although *splitting* is a term that came into popular usage as one of the principal defense mechanisms of patients with borderline personality disorder, the definition has since been expanded through popular usage to connote an interpersonal process as well as an intrapsychic mechanism. Specifically, *splitting* tends to be used to describe situations in which staff members involved in treatment settings such as inpatient units or day hospitals are polarized against each other in their views of the patient's treatment needs. In this broadened usage, transference-countertransference dimensions of patient-staff interactions related to the mechanism of projective identification are clearly implied. Moreover, because a hostile or aggressive undercurrent is often associated with splitting, the term has developed a pejorative connotation. For example, nurses, activities therapists, psychiatrists, psychologists, and other mental health professionals commonly refer to a patient as a "splitter" in the same tone of voice they would describe a hardened criminal. Similarly, when a disagreement occurs between two treaters involved in the hospitalization of a patient with borderline personality disorder, one is likely to observe to the other: "The patient is splitting us."

Such glib pronouncements may at once ease the tension between the treaters and appear to explain the disagreement by "blaming" the patient. However, the use of the term *splitting* may or may not be accurate in the context in which it is heard. As one unfortunate consequence of its popularization, the concept has been overused and applied to a variety of situations that threaten to rob the term of its specific meaning. *Splitting* has become a wastebasket of sorts that serves as a repository for a wide range of behaviors and experiences involving various forms of manipulation, transference-countertransference phenomena, and virtually all varieties of disagreements among staff members. In this chapter we discuss a more specific conceptualization of splitting that both defines a specific conceptualization that has implications for the management of countertransference and differentiates the term from other clinical phenomena with which it may be confused (Gabbard 1989).

Developmental Origins of Splitting

A number of authors (Freedman 1981; Lichtenberg and Slapp 1973; Lustman 1977; Pruyser 1975) have commented on the wide and varied usage of the splitting concept. The multiple connotations of the term, stemming from diverse theoretical underpinnings, have even led some to advocate abandonment of the term (Pruyser 1975). For the most part, however, the general consensus is that the key notion involves maintaining contradictory aspects of intrapsychic experience separate. Moreover, most authors would agree that splitting is both a normal developmental mode of organizing the infant's intrapsychic experience and a defense mechanism that ultimately arises from this mode.

Although Freud seemed to prefer the defense of repression to that of splitting, references to splitting of the ego are scattered throughout his papers (Grotstein 1981). Particularly toward the latter part of his career, references to the phenomenon became increasingly common. In his 1927 paper on fetishism, Freud described two states of mind coexisting side by side although each was associated with an idea that seemed incompatible with the other. By the time of his death, Freud had become convinced that splitting was virtually a universal feature of human psychopathology that derived from infancy and persisted in neurotic as well as in psychotic and fetishist patients (Freud 1940/1964a, 1940/1964b).

Although classical analysts for the most part failed to see the value of Freud's concept, Melanie Klein (1946/1975) viewed splitting as essential to understanding the infant's early anxieties. Convinced that life constituted a struggle between the life and death instincts, Klein viewed splitting as the cornerstone of emotional survival in the first several months of life. Splitting allows the infant to separate good from bad, pleasure from unpleasure, and love from hate to preserve positively colored experiences, affects, and self-representations in a safely isolated mental compartment, free from contamination by their negative counterparts.

We can best illustrate the developmental basis of splitting by examining the infant's feeding experience. A prototype of loving positive experience is formed during periods when the infant is nursing (Freud 1905/1953). This prototype includes a positive experience of the self (the nursing infant); a positive experience of the object (the attentive, caretaking mother); and a positive affective experience (pleasure, satiation). When hunger returns and the infant's mother is not immediately available, a prototype of negative experience occurs, including a negative experience of the self (the frustrated, demanding infant); an inattentive, frustrating object (the unavailable mother); and a negative affective experience of anger and perhaps terror. Indeed, the infant's mother is both nurturing and frustrating and therefore the fundamental source of splitting (Mahler 1968). Ultimately, these two experiences are internalized as two opposing sets of object relationships consisting of a self-representation, an object-representation, and an affect linking the two (Fairbairn 1940/1952, 1944/1952; Gabbard 1986; Masterson and Rinsley 1975; Ogden 1983; Rinsley 1977).

The internalization of the infant's mother, usually referred to as introjection (Schafer 1968), begins with the physical sensations associated with the mother's presence during nursing, but does not become meaningful until a boundary between inner and outer has developed. Isolated images of the mother gradually coalesce into an enduring mental representation of her around the 16th month of life (Sandler and Rosenblatt 1962). At the same time an enduring self-representation forms, first as a body-representation and later as a compilation of sensations and experiences perceived as belonging to the infant. Representations in these early stages are necessarily rudimentary because of the limitations of the cognitive and perceptual faculties of the infant (Lustman 1977).

The positively colored or "good" object-representation begins as a hallucinatory wish fulfillment stemming from the hungry infant's longing for the mother (Schafer 1968) and is later transformed into an internal presence as the infant's cognitive perceptual apparatus develops. A major motivating force in the introjection of the positive, loving aspects of the mother seems to be the infant's fear of losing the mother (Schafer 1968). The reasons for the introjection or "taking in" of the negative, "bad" aspects of the mother are more complex. Possible motivating factors include the fantasy of controlling the object by containing it within oneself (Segal 1964), gaining a sense of mastery through repeated traumatic experiences with the object (Schafer 1968), and a preference for a bad object over no object at all (Schafer 1968). Clinical experience suggests that intense attachment to an internalized hostile object may also be connected with a yearning for a more positive relationship with the object (Meissner 1981). Furthermore, the object that has been introjected does not necessarily correlate with the real external object. For example, a mother who is unavailable to feed her infant on demand may simply be occupied with an older sibling, even though she is experienced and introjected by the infant as hostile, rejecting, and unavailable.

Even before the self- and object-representations are firmly established, one can observe forerunners of splitting. The good, loving experiences are kept separate from the bad, terrifying experiences to preserve a safe climate for feeding. Nursing would be disrupted if negative images of the unavailable mother were allowed to intrude. As boundaries between the inside and outside develop and images coalesce into representations, negative aspects of the self- and object-representations threaten to destroy the positive aspects. Hence, splitting is maintained as an active defensive process to keep good separated from bad (Kernberg 1967). The introjects resulting from this process are often referred to as "part objects" as a way of acknowledging that they lack the "whole" quality of more mature introjects, which are characterized by a mixture of positive and negative qualities.

Splitting is enhanced by projection, which involves unconsciously attributing the bad qualities to another person while all good qualities remain within, thus effecting a further separation of the polarized aspects. Positive or good attributes of the self- or object-representations may also be projected to keep them at a safe distance from the bad within (Segal 1964). In this manner splitting serves to bring order to the infant's early chaotic experience (Freedman 1981; Lichtenberg and Slapp 1973; Lustman 1977; Ogden 1986). Furthermore, by managing danger in a way that is necessary for the infant's emotional survival, it constitutes the original paradigm of intrapsychic defense (Lustman 1977; Odgen 1986).

Splitting is best understood as a universal mechanism growing out of normal development. Although it may operate across a broad spectrum of diagnostic categories (Freedman 1981; Perry and Cooper 1986; Rangell 1982), much of the term's popularity is derived from Kernberg's (1967, 1975) notion that splitting is the key defensive operation involved in the borderline personality disorder. He described splitting as an active process of keeping contradictory introjects and affects separate, resulting in the following clinical manifestations: 1) alternating expressions of contradictory behaviors and attitudes, which the patient regards with lack of concern and bland denial; 2) selective lack of impulse control; 3) compartmentalization of all persons in the patient's environment into all-good and all-bad camps; and 4) coexistence of contradictory self-representations that alternate in their dominance from day to day and from hour to hour.

The studies of normal and pathological mother-infant dyads by Mahler and colleagues (1975) provide some observational data to bolster Kernberg's (1967, 1975) view that the developmental fixation in patients with borderline personality disorder occurs at a point in childhood before the integration of good and bad part objects into an ambivalently regarded whole object. Mahler and her colleagues supplied empirical evidence to suggest that such integration does not occur until the child achieves object constancy at age 2½ or 3 years. They reasoned that the intense separation anxiety typical of the patient with borderline personality disorder is connected to this failure of object constancy, which leaves the patient without an integrated whole object-representation that can provide soothing functions in the absence of an actual parent.

This developmental model of the origins of splitting, which is largely based on Klein, Mahler, and Kernberg, has been challenged by the infant observation studies of Stern (1985). Although Stern agreed that splitting is a universal experience, he suggested that an infant is not capable of such advanced symbolic thinking. He also regarded the compartmentalization of the infant's experience into a dichotomy of "good" and "bad" as an oversimplified version of the feeding experience. His observations suggested that infants have a variety of different experiences with nursing that form a gradient of pleasurable and unpleasurable experience. He also challenged the view that the split between good and bad affective states precedes the ability to differentiate self from other. No clear sequence of dichotomies emerged from his infant observations, and Stern concluded that the ability to distinguish self and object emerges simultaneously with the differentiation between positively and negatively charged affective states.

Another problem pointed out by Stern (1985) is the glib equation between what is "good" and what is "pleasurable," on the one hand, and what is "bad" and what is "unpleasurable," on the other hand. He noted that goodness and badness connote a moral dimension, and he stressed that infants are not capable of making such complex symbolic judgments about the intentions of caretakers who are providing pleasurable or unpleasurable experiences. Stern argued that infants are capable of such subtleties in their thinking only at the more mature stage of intersubjective relatedness, not during the first year of life. He observed the grouping of interpersonal experiences into pleasurable and unpleasurable categories or "hedonic clusters," but he did not agree that these clusters are responsible for the compartmentalization or splitting of all interpersonal experiences along lines of pleasure and unpleasure. Stern's view of development emphasized that infants initially encounter and internalize *reality* and only later begin distorting reality based on defensive needs. His view is in stark contrast with that of Melanie Klein (1946/1975), who believed that fantasies were operative from the first year of life and were highly influential in the internalization of object relationships.

Although Klein's (1946/1975) attribution of sophisticated adult symbolic capacities to the infant is consensually viewed as no longer tenable, other infant investigators do not entirely share Stern's (1985) view. Parens (1979a, 1979b, 1991), for example, noted behavior suggestive of splitting from age 9 months on. In his studies of the development of hostility and aggression, Parens argued that excessive degrees of unpleasurable experience tend to generate hostile destructiveness. When the child cannot cope with hostile, destructive feelings toward its caretaker, the child begins to develop split object-representations as a defensive maneuver. However, Parens also stressed that stable, hostile, destructive affect attached to self and object experiences does not appear to become internalized until about midway through the second year of life.

Although all infant observation studies are hampered by the methodological necessity of inferring internal experience from externally observed behavior, most data collected point to the consolidation of split self-object-affect units somewhere between 18 months and 3 years of age. The popular usage of "good" and "bad" to describe these units is an unfortunate oversimplification in the literature. A variety of other adjectives are needed to capture the complexity of the interpersonal relationships that are internalized and the affects associated with them.

A number of authors (Adler 1985; Gabbard 1986; Kernberg 1967, 1975; Klein 1946/1975; Odgen 1979, 1983, 1986; Shapiro et al. 1977) have commented on the intimate relationship between splitting and projective identification. Ogden (1986) noted that when an infant's positive view of the mother is threatened by a diametrically opposed perception, the latter can be projected externally as a way of separating the endangering object-representation from the endangered one. In this manner, projective identification develops as an interpersonal elaboration of the intrapsychic splitting process.

In summary, splitting and projective identification are two interrelated mechanisms that provide a basic mode of organizing experience from early in life. The loved mother can be separated from the feared and hated mother; the hating self of the infant can be compartmentalized apart from the loving self. These mechanisms

allow the infant to feed safely without fear of intrusion from negative self- or object-representations. These operations prevent the
good from being destroyed by the bad and provide an opportunity
for the infant to experience disturbing aspects of the self and others
at a distance until he or she is more psychologically ready for the
task of integration.

Splitting in Settings Involving Multiple Treaters

In settings involving multiple treaters, such as inpatient units and
day hospitals, the combination of splitting and projective identification can become a highly disruptive force in the milieu. Splitting in
the hospital has been well described in a number of papers on the
intense countertransference evoked by treatment-resistant patients
with borderline personality disorder (Burnham 1966; Gabbard
1986; Main 1957). Staff members find themselves assuming highly
polarized positions and defending those positions against one another with a vehemence that is out of proportion to the importance
of the issue. The patient has presented one self-representation to
one group of treaters and another self-representation to another
group of treaters (Burnham 1966; Cohen 1957; Gabbard 1986;
Searles 1965). Through projective identification, each self-
representation evokes a corresponding reaction in the treater that
can be understood as an unconscious identification with the projected internal object of the patient. The transference-countertransference paradigm produced by one self-object constellation
may be dramatically different from that produced by another. This
discrepancy may first manifest itself in a staff meeting where the
patient is being discussed. One group of staff members becomes
puzzled by the description they are hearing and may ask, "Are we
talking about the same patient?"

Full-blown splitting of this variety illustrates the time-honored
notion that patients recapitulate their own internal object world in
the hospital milieu. Various treaters become unconsciously identified with the patient's various internal objects and play out roles in

a drama that is written by the patient's unconscious. Moreover, because of the element of control inherent in projective identification, there is often an obligatory quality to the treaters' responses. They feel compelled to behave "like someone else." If projective identification were not involved, the purely intrapsychic splitting that would result would cause little disturbance in the staff group. Nor would the staff group view the process as an example of splitting, since they would probably not feel polarized and angry toward one another.

The splitting that occurs in settings with multiple treaters represents a special case in which both intrapsychic and interpersonal splitting are taking place simultaneously (Gabbard 1989; Hamilton 1988). The interpersonal aspects of splitting that occur in staff groups clearly parallel the intrapsychic splitting occurring in the patient. Projective identification is the vehicle that converts intrapsychic splitting into interpersonal splitting.

As we noted in Chapter 1, staff members who are singled out as recipients of the patient's projected internal objects are not randomly selected. More often than not, patients with borderline personality disorder have an uncanny ability to detect preexisting latent conflict among various staff members, and their projections may be guided accordingly. A vignette from an actual case illustrates this pattern.

> Ms. K was a 29-year-old patient with borderline personality disorder admitted to a psychiatric unit after a suicide attempt. She had a long history of sexual abuse, self-mutilation, and suicide attempts. One week after admission to the unit, she was in the day area when one of the nurses noticed that blood was dripping from under the sleeve of her blouse. The nurse rolled up the sleeve and found three longitudinal lacerations that required suturing. Later that day in a staff meeting, the nurse ventilated her anger at Ms. K by saying, "She is such a sneak! She told me that she had no razors or other sharp objects in her room. She looked me straight in the eye and lied to me. All the time she was saying that, she knew a razor was in her light fixture, hidden there so she could cut herself."
>
> The psychologist on the treatment team immediately jumped

to the patient's defense, pointedly saying to the nurse, "I think you need to look at your own contribution to the situation. The patient asked to speak to you, and you told her you didn't have time. She was reaching out and trying to communicate instead of turning to self-mutilation, and you let her down. I can see why she cut herself."

The nurse in turn lashed back at the psychologist: "That's easy for you to say. You sit in your office drinking coffee and writing test reports all day. You're not with the patients 8 hours a day. You don't know what it's like to have five different patients demanding something from you at one time. It's impossible to meet all those demands."

The psychologist then defended his point of view: "Look, Ms. K is the victim of an unbelievably horrible background. She was sexually abused by her stepfather for 8 years. Her mother might as well have been completely absent from the picture. She needs to feel that she is special. She needs to know that staff are there to respond to her special needs so that she will feel validated as a person. You can't just treat her like every other patient."

The nurse retorted, "You always get into this position of saying that we need to individualize treatment more. I don't think you realize how difficult that is. Also, I don't think you realize how nasty and manipulative this patient is. I think you got suckered in by her during the testing. What she needs is to be treated like everyone else!"

This glimpse of an emotionally charged moment in the treatment of Ms. K illustrates how different staff members become the repository for different aspects of the patient's internal world. One can infer that in the privacy of the psychologist's office, Ms. K presented a particular self-representation that evoked a complementary object-representation in the psychologist. As she told the psychologist her long history of victimization, the psychologist fell into the complementary role of the idealized and omnipotent rescuer who would give the patient the special treatment she longed for. When Ms. K returned to the unit after her testing, she recognized that she was one patient among many, and to obtain the attention she felt she required, she raised her level of stridency and demandingness to an obnoxious degree. This behavior—emblematic of a different self-representation—coerced a different complementary object response in the nurse.

Staff members are therefore polarized into thinking their own point of view is correct. At such moments, a level-headed leader of the treatment team is needed to point out that who is right and who is wrong is not the issue. Both staff members are identifying legitimate aspects of the patient's internal world. Moreover, if they view the relationship with the psychologist as therapeutic while they see the relationship with the nurse as countertherapeutic, they have missed the point. The therapeutic relationship must be viewed as an overarching whole composed of fragments played out in individual relationships (Gabbard 1992). Hence staff meetings in inpatient work serve a container function, where the projected fragments are identified and integrated into a coherent picture of the patient's psyche. After the polarized treaters work through their differences in the context of a staff meeting, Ms. K will have a better chance of integrating her internal fragments.

This case example demonstrates how splitting and projective identification do not occur in a vacuum. Ms. K clearly picked out individuals who conveniently fit the internal object-relationship paradigms assigned to them. As several authors (Adler 1985; Burnham 1966; Shapiro et al. 1977) noted, the assignment of internal object projections to staff members is often based on a kernel of reality. This vignette also reflects Burnham's observation that the cleavage is usually between those treaters who emphasize the administrative frame of reference (what is good for the group) versus those who emphasize an individualistic frame of reference based on what is good for an individual patient (Burnham 1966).

Although not the case in this particular example, perhaps the most common variety of splitting found in the treatment of borderline patients is the idealization of the psychotherapist as an "all-good" object associated with the devaluation of the milieu staff as insensitive, punitive, and "all bad." This form of splitting may be intensified by the tendency of many borderline patients in psychotherapy sessions to omit information deriving from day-to-day unit activities because they are focusing exclusively on childhood memories and transference material (Adler 1985; Kernberg 1984). The psychotherapist, then, has no awareness of the problematic interactions on the unit and is caught by surprise when nursing staff or day hospital workers bring them up. Similarly, milieu staff have no awareness of some of the childhood traumas that the patient is relating only to the therapist.

Adler (1985) noted that the hospital staff may actually exclude the psychotherapist from the process of treatment planning as a result of this form of splitting. In this manner the unit staff may consolidate the alliance with one another by projecting badness and incompetence outside the unit group onto the psychotherapist. If this process goes on unchecked, the unit staff and the psychotherapist find it impossible to reconcile their differences and meet each other halfway. Just like the patient's internal objects, they cannot be integrated. The regressive power of groups is well-known and may result in the use of splitting and projective identification in otherwise well-integrated professionals (Bion 1961; Kernberg 1984; Oldham and Russakoff 1987).

When a staff group reaches this point of fragmentation, all too often the patient is blamed for attempting to "divide and conquer" (Rinsley 1980). What is often forgotten under these circumstances is that splitting is an unconscious process that patients use automatically to maintain their emotional survival. We do not generally blame patients for other defense mechanisms. The unique issue in splitting seems to be the treaters' perception that the patient is being consciously and maliciously destructive. An empathic frame of reference is useful to remind staff members that patients use splitting as an attempt to ward off destructiveness and to protect themselves from being destroyed.

To summarize, splitting in settings with multiple treaters involves four primary features (Gabbard 1989). First, the process occurs at an unconscious level. Second, the patient perceives different staff members in dramatically different ways, based on projections of the patient's internal object-representations, and treats each staff member differentially according to those projections. Third, staff members react to the patient, through projective identification, as though they actually were the projected aspects of the patient. Fourth, as a result, treaters assume highly polarized positions in staff discussions about the patient and defend those positions with extraordinary vehemence.

Although the focus here has been on multiple treater settings such as inpatient units and day hospitals, splitting is a potential problem even when only two treaters are involved. Perhaps the most common dual-clinician situation is a division of labor between a psychotherapist and a pharmacotherapist. Therapists who "split off" the medication issues from the psychotherapy as though they exist outside the realm of dynamic understanding do so at their own peril (Waldinger and Frank 1989). Pharmacologic agents are frequently viewed by borderline patients as transitional objects, as shortcuts allowing them to avoid psychotherapy, as signs that the therapist is abandoning them, and as an indication of psychotherapeutic failure. Regardless of whether the therapist or an adjunctive pharmacotherapist is doing the prescribing, the patient's fantasies about the meanings of the medication must be an active part of the psychotherapeutic process.

Variants of Splitting

The features enumerated here serve to distinguish splitting involving both intrapsychic and interpersonal dimensions from variants that also occur commonly in multiple-treater settings.

Intrapsychic Splitting

Splitting, as already described, has a powerful interpersonal aspect due to the associated projective identification process. However, when splitting occurs without projective identification, it may remain a purely intrapsychic phenomenon.

> Mr. J, a 44-year-old attorney, appeared an assertive and hypermasculine presence in the courtroom. At night, however, he liked to dress in women's clothing and think of himself as an elegant lady. These two contradictory self-representations presented little conflict for the patient, who regarded them with bland denial

by saying simply, "I'm a multifaceted person." Both of these dimensions emerged in his hospital treatment, but neither produced intense countertransference reactions in the treaters.

Some patients with borderline personality disorder display alternating self-representations to different staff members, but they simply do not evoke corresponding object responses. Hence, no significant interpersonal dimension is activated, and staff members are not likely to engage in vociferous disagreements of the kind seen in splitting associated with projective identification. Also, even in cases when object responses *are* evoked, they may diminish over time as staff members begin to understand the process. What begins as an interpersonal phenomenon may evolve into a purely intrapsychic one.

Manipulation

Patients with borderline personality disorder are frequently referred to as manipulators, and their manipulative behavior is frequently called splitting. Because patients who suffer from borderline pathology live in constant dread of abandonment, they often display an inordinate need to control the behavior of others, thereby reassuring themselves that they are not vulnerable to the whims of those around them. Such patients will often go from one staff member to another trying to get the attention they think they need. Similarly, they may make mild self-destructive gestures or engage in other acting-out behaviors that are designed to ensure that treaters will pay attention to them. To elicit the response they wish to receive, they will flatter, cajole, coax, seduce, or otherwise coerce the treatment staff.

> Ms. I, a 20-year-old college student, felt like no one on the hospital treatment staff was paying sufficient attention to her. In group meetings she would assert that all the other patients on the team received more "staff time" than she did. As a way of extracting more interaction time from the nursing staff, she would frequently bring up somatic complaints. One evening she went to four different nurses with the same physical complaint. When she did not receive

the attention she desired from one nurse, she would seek out another nurse, hoping that this one would satisfy her needs. After going through all four staff members without success, she gave up and went to her room, where it was reported that she was sulking. In the staff meeting the next day, one of the nurses reported that she felt Ms. I was "splitting" staff by seeking out other opinions when she wasn't getting what she wanted from the first nurse she approached.

Although this behavior was called splitting, each staff member, in fact, was viewed and treated the same. Moreover, the process was operating at a largely conscious level. (Ms. I later admitted that she was using the complaint to get attention.) Finally, although there was some projective identification, as evidenced by the intense anger the nursing staff felt toward the patient, the nursing staff did not feel split into different camps as a result of differing identifications, nor did they have any substantial disagreement about what the patient was doing. On the contrary, the treatment team was considerably united in how they perceived the patient. In other words, one internal object-representation was consistently being projected in all interactions.

Unfortunately, when patients are seen as manipulative, they are often blamed for the behavior rather than viewed in an empathic context. The knowledge that Ms. I had a conscious wish for attention should not have obscured the unconscious internal object relationship that was being played out as well. An aspect of the self was yearning for a particular object response. Adler (1985) pointed out that some manipulation is largely unconscious and has an adaptive function in that the patient keeps from being alone. If the treatment staff keep this perspective in mind, they can gain greater mastery over countertransference reactions.

Lying

Although linked in some ways to manipulation, lying is more consciously exploitative and ruthless in its intent. Patients with borderline personality disorder with prominent antisocial features are obviously more likely to engage in deception, and their dishonesty presents a whole array of treatment problems. Since lying can often set one staff member against another, this behavior is often erroneously viewed as splitting.

> Mr. H, a 29-year-old drug abuser, was in extended hospital treatment for a variety of problems stemming from dysfunction in relationships and job situations and failure to respond to short-term interventions designed to help him with his drug abuse. Part of the structure established on the unit was for him to open all letters in front of staff members because he had been receiving drugs through the mail. One evening when Mr. H received his mail, he informed Ms. P, a nurse who was preparing to observe Mr. H's letter opening, that he no longer needed to follow this element of his structure because his doctor had told him that such observation had outlived its usefulness. The next day Ms. P angrily confronted Mr. H's doctor and told him that such decisions should be discussed with all staff members in team meetings. She went on to say that she resented the doctor's unilateral decision making on this issue because she felt it was still necessary. Mr. H's doctor categorically denied that he had made any such statement to Mr. H. When the doctor and Ms. P went to Mr. H together and confronted him, the patient acknowledged that he had lied.

Although lying may turn staff members against one another, the cleavage does not result from the patient's alternating self-representations presented differentially to different staff members. The process is conscious and is far more malicious than the unconscious splitting process.

Staff Disagreement

All disagreements among staff members on a treatment team are not the result of splitting. Staff members working together will have a variety of different treatment philosophies regarding such matters as the use of structure, limit setting, gratification versus frustration of transference wishes, and the optimal level of staff control versus patient autonomy, to name just a few. Although these preexisting differences may serve as the nidus for splitting maneuvers by the patient with borderline personality disorder, many other instances occur in which staff members simply disagree because of differing philosophies.

In treatment team meetings, staff members commonly blame the patient for these philosophical disagreements when one member might say, "The patient must be splitting us. This says more about the patient than it does about us." This kind of statement lets the treaters off the hook. They do not have to attempt to resolve their differences. Instead, they can talk about the patient's tendency to engage in splitting.

The differentiation of staff disagreement from splitting is complex. The intensity with which positions are defended may be a useful index of the presence of splitting. When mere philosophical differences are present, one person usually retains some ability to listen to others and has some empathic appreciation for the differing point of view. In the throes of splitting and projective identification, however, each person has become so polarized that no one has the ability to see any value at all in the opposition, and the discussion frequently deteriorates into personal attacks.

This index is not foolproof, however, because group dynamics may result in splitting and polarization independent of the patient's influence. These phenomena are particularly likely to occur when the work task of the staff group becomes unclear or derailed and when staff members are feeling demoralized (Bion 1961). Differentiation of these group phenomena from patient-induced polarization may be possible by determining if the group differences occur along lines that parallel the patient's internal object world.

The Management of Splitting

Any discussion of how to manage splitting in settings with multiple treaters must begin with Burnham's (1966) caveat that the complete prevention of splitting is neither possible nor desirable. As is the case with other defense mechanisms, splitting provides a safety valve that protects the patient from what is perceived as overwhelming danger. The process will develop regardless of what preventive measures are implemented. The essential point here is that splitting must be continuously monitored by treatment staff to prevent it from destroying the patient's treatment, devastating the morale of the staff, and irreparably damaging certain interstaff relationships. Cases of serious psychiatric morbidity and staff resignations have resulted from such situations (Burnham 1966; Main 1957).

The importance of education cannot be overemphasized. All mental health professionals should be thoroughly conversant with the concept of splitting and its variants. If staff members cannot recognize splitting when it develops, the management of the situation may be hopeless. Clinical directors of psychiatric units or day hospitals must establish a cultural norm in which countertransference feelings are viewed as an acceptable part of the treatment process and as containing valuable information about the patient (Gabbard 1986). In discussions of countertransference, staff members can be encouraged to work toward containing projected aspects of the patient rather than acting on them. Intense feelings toward patients should be viewed as useful material for discussion and supervision rather than forbidden reactions that must be concealed from one's supervisor. The mechanism of splitting can be explained to unit staff members so that they can avoid exploiting a split by not accepting idealization and not colluding with the devaluation of other staff members (Adler 1973; Shapiro et al. 1977). Monitoring the countertransference tendencies of staff members to project aspects of themselves onto the patient is also crucial.

Education is only a beginning, however. Regular and frequent staff meetings that include the patient's psychotherapist should be a part of the weekly routine. A spirit of open communication about differences should be established and monitored by the treatment team. About 40 years ago Stanton and Schwartz (1954) persuasively demonstrated the prophylactic value of ferreting out covert staff disagreements and making them overt. Psychotherapists must view themselves as part of the treatment team and ally themselves with administrative decisions made by the team. Rigid adherence to concerns about confidentiality may feed right into the patient's splitting tendencies.

One major goal in the treatment of patients with borderline

personality disorder is the integration of split self- and object-representations. Although interpretation of the splitting mechanism is useful in helping patients achieve more moderated and realistic views of themselves and others, rarely is interpretation alone sufficient to mend the cleavage that occurs at the group level. Interpretations made to the patient are best viewed as adjuncts to other staff interventions and interactions. Corresponding to the psychotherapist's approach to the internal world of the patient, integration and moderation of the *external* objects are the goals of staff intervention.

To this end, joint meetings of the staff member identified with the bad object, the treater identified with the good object, and the patient, to discuss frankly the patient's perception of what is going on are often useful. This arrangement makes the patient's polarized views more difficult to maintain; both treaters are seen as acting humanely and reasonably. Moreover, treaters ordinarily become less polarized and move toward middle ground when they are faced with this situation. The very separateness demanded by the splitting mechanism is undermined. Although this may temporarily increase the patient's anxiety, the message is also conveyed that negative feelings can be contained within interpersonal relationships without disastrous consequences.

When the situation is so emotionally charged that the participants are not willing to meet, an objective consultant can be brought in as a mediator in the discussion (Gabbard 1986). The mediator can perform the role of an observing ego for the group and thereby encourage those individuals involved with the splitting to identify with that function, much as Shapiro and colleagues (1977) described the function of the psychotherapist when meeting with borderline adolescents and their families.

These meetings presuppose a recognition by all parties that a splitting process is going on. Such acknowledgment constitutes a major step toward successful management of splitting. Ordinarily, staff members experience considerable reluctance to see themselves involved in splitting. When a special meeting is called to discuss the staff dynamics surrounding a particular patient, treaters may show strong resistance because they feel that such a meeting will make the patient too special (Burnham 1966). If the patient's psychotherapist is involved in the split, he or she may be willing to attend the staff meeting but will come with a different agenda. If idealized by the patient, the therapist is especially likely to assume the condescending position of educating the staff about their countertransference reactions and about the dynamics of the patient so they will understand the patient as well as the psychotherapist does. The psychotherapist's implicit message in this situation is that by understanding the patient, the other staff members will stop blaming the patient. Rather than seeing the staff meeting as a productive way to discuss a splitting process, the psychotherapist's view is that he or she is right while everyone else is wrong. Being idealized may be so gratifying that the therapist does not wish to examine the idealization (Finell 1985) nor consider it a part of the patient's defensive process. This approach will, of course, infuriate the other staff even further and widen the split.

When a staff meeting is called to discuss potential splitting, the parties should approach one another with the assumption that each is a reasonable and competent clinician who cares about the patient's welfare. When this approach works, the group feels that each staff member has brought forth a piece of the puzzle so that the whole is more clearly seen (Burnham 1966). However, some splits seem irreparable; just as the internal objects of the patient cannot be integrated, neither can the external objects reconcile with one another. If the therapist is cast in the role of the devalued object, such stalemates occasionally end with the other staff members recommending a new therapist (Adler 1985).

The earlier the process is discovered, the less entrenched it will be and the more amenable to change. Certain warning signals should be continuously monitored in staff meetings: 1) when a treater is uncharacteristically punitive toward a patient, 2) when a treater is unusually indulgent, 3) when one treater repeatedly defends a patient against critical comments from other staff members, and 4) when staff members feel that only they can understand the patient.

When staff members can swallow their pride and accept that they may be involved in an unconscious identification with projected aspects of the patient, they can begin to empathize with other staff members' feelings and perspectives. This willingness to consider someone else's point of view can lead to collaborative work on the patient's behalf that results in marked improvement in the splitting process. The patient's internal split often begins to mend at the same time the treatment team's external cleavage heals (Gabbard 1986). These parallel developments may be understood as the third step of projective identification—the previously split-off and projected object-representations of the patient are contained and modified by the treaters and then reintrojected in modified form by the patient in a meaningful interpersonal context. By approaching their own differences in good faith, treaters provide an atmosphere in the milieu where good experiences predominate over bad ones, an essential condition to facilitate the integration of love and hate in the patient.

Summary

In settings with multiple treaters, the combination of splitting and projective identification can divide the staff into "good" and "bad" groups from the patient's point of view. Splitting in such settings involves four primary features. First, the process occurs at an unconscious level. Second, the patient perceives different staff members in dramatically different ways, based on projections of the patient's internal object-representations, and treats each staff member differentially, according to those projections. Third, staff members react to the patient, through projective identification, as though they actually were the projected aspects of the patient. Fourth, as a result, treaters assume highly polarized positions in staff discussions about the patient and defend those positions with extraordinary vehemence.

The first step in the management of splitting in multiple-treater settings is to recognize it for what it is. Staff education is essential, so that all the mental health professionals involved in the treatment have an understanding of the mechanisms of splitting and projective identification. Regular and frequent staff meetings that include all members of the treatment team are also an important part of a weekly routine. If one key member of the treatment team is not present, the potential exists for greater distortion without the possibility of hearing all points of view. Joint meetings of the "bad" object and the "good" object with the patient are often useful as well. In situations of extreme staff disruption, an objective consultant may be brought in as a mediator. Finally, all staff members should be aware of warning signals that suggest the development of a splitting process within the milieu.

References

Adler G: Hospital treatment of borderline patients. Am J Psychiatry 130:32–35, 1973

Adler G: Borderline Psychopathology and Its Treatment. New York, Jason Aronson, 1985

Bion WR: Experiences in Groups and Other Papers. New York, Basic Books, 1961

Burnham DL: The special problem patient: victim or agent of splitting? Psychiatry 29:105–122, 1966

Cohen RA: Some relations between staff tensions and the psychotherapeutic process, in The Patient and the Mental Hospital: Contributions of Research in the Science of Social Behavior. Edited by Greenblatt M, Levinson DJ, Williams RH. Glencoe, IL, Free Press, 1957, pp 301–308

Fairbairn WRD: Schizoid factors in the personality (1940), in Psychoanalytic Studies of the Personality. London, Routledge & Kegan Paul, 1952, pp 3–27

Fairbairn WRD: Endopsychic structure considered in terms of object-relationships (1944), in Psychoanalytic Studies of the Personality. London, Routledge & Kegan Paul, 1952, pp 82–136

Finell JS: Narcissistic problems in analysts. Int J Psychoanal 66:433–445, 1985

Freedman N: Varieties of splitting, in Object and Self: A Developmental Approach. Edited by Tuttman S, Kaye C, Zimmerman M. New York, International Universities Press, 1981, pp 267–289

Freud S: Three essays on the theory of sexuality (1905), in The Standard Edition of the Complete Psychological Works of Sigmund Freud, Vol 7. Translated and edited by Strachey J. London, Hogarth Press, 1953, pp 123–245

Freud S: Fetishism (1927), in The Standard Edition of the Complete Psychological Works of Sigmund Freud, Vol 21. Translated and edited by Strachey J. London, Hogarth Press, 1961, pp 147–157

Freud S: An outline of psycho-analysis (1940), in The Standard Edition of the Complete Psychological Works of Sigmund Freud, Vol 23. Translated and edited by Strachey J. London, Hogarth Press, 1964a, pp 139–207

Freud S: Splitting of the ego in the process of defence (1940), in The Standard Edition of the Complete Psychological Works of Sigmund Freud, Vol 23. Translated and edited by Strachey J. London, Hogarth Press, 1964b, pp 271–278

Gabbard GO: The treatment of the "special" patient in a psychoanalytic hospital. International Review of Psychoanalysis 13:333–347, 1986

Gabbard GO: Splitting in hospital treatment. Am J Psychiatry 146:444–451, 1989

Gabbard GO: The therapeutic relationship in psychiatric hospital treatment. Bull Menninger Clin 56:4–19, 1992

Grotstein JS: Splitting and Projective Identification. New York, Jason Aronson, 1981

Hamilton NG: Self and Others: Object Relations Theory in Practice. Northvale, NJ, Jason Aronson, 1988

Kernberg OF: Borderline personality organization. J Am Psychoanal Assoc 15:641–685, 1967

Kernberg OF: Borderline Conditions and Pathological Narcissism. New York, Jason Aronson, 1975

Kernberg OF: Severe Personality Disorders: Psychotherapeutic Strategies. New Haven, CT, Yale University Press, 1984

Klein M: Notes on some schizoid mechanisms (1946), in Envy and Gratitude and Other Works, 1946–1963. New York, Delacorte, 1975

Lichtenberg JD, Slapp JW: Notes on the concept of splitting and the defense mechanism of the splitting of representations. J Am Psychoanal Assoc 21:772–787, 1973

Lustman J: On splitting. Psychoanal Study Child 32:119–154, 1977

Mahler MS: On Human Symbiosis and the Vicissitudes of Individuation, Vol 1: Infantile Psychosis. New York, International Universities Press, 1968

Mahler MS, Pine F, Bergman A: The Psychological Birth of the Human Infant: Symbiosis and Individuation. New York, Basic Books, 1975

Main TF: The ailment. Br J Med Psychol 30:129–145, 1957

Masterson JF, Rinsley DB: The borderline syndrome: the role of the mother in the genesis and psychic structure of the borderline personality. Int J Psychoanal 56:163–177, 1975

Meissner WW: Internalization in Psychoanalysis. New York, International Universities Press, 1981

Ogden TH: On projective identification. Int J Psychoanal 60:357–373, 1979

Ogden TH: The concept of internal object relations. Int J Psychoanal 64:227–241, 1983

Ogden TH: The Matrix of the Mind: Object Relations and the Psychoanalytic Dialogue. Northvale, NJ, Jason Aronson, 1986

Oldham JM, Russakoff LM: Dynamic Therapy in Brief Hospitalization. Northvale, NJ, Jason Aronson, 1987

Parens H: Developmental considerations of ambivalence: part 2 of an exploration of the relations of instinctual drives and the symbiosis-separation-individuation process. Psychoanal Study Child 34:385–420, 1979a

Parens H: The Development of Aggression in Early Childhood. New York, Jason Aronson, 1979b

Parens H: A view of the development of hostility in early life. J Am Psychoanal Assoc 39 (suppl):75–108, 1991

Perry JC, Cooper SH: A preliminary report on defenses and conflicts associated with borderline personality disorder. J Am Psychoanal Assoc 34:863–893, 1986

Pruyser PW: What splits in splitting? a scrutiny of the concept of splitting in psychoanalysis and psychiatry. Bull Menninger Clin 39:1–46, 1975

Rangell L: The self in psychoanalytic theory. J Am Psychoanal Assoc 30:863–891, 1982

Rinsley DB: An object relations view of borderline personality, in Borderline Personality Disorders. Edited by Hartocollis P. New York, International Universities Press, 1977, pp 47–70

Rinsley DB: Treatment of the Severely Disturbed Adolescent. New York, Jason Aronson, 1980

Sandler J, Rosenblatt B: The concept of the representational world. Psychoanal Study Child 17:128–145, 1962

Schafer R: Aspects of Internalization. New York, International Universities Press, 1968

Searles H: Collected Papers on Schizophrenia and Related Subjects. New York, International Universities Press, 1965

Segal H: An Introduction to the Work of Melanie Klein. New York, Basic Books, 1964

Shapiro ER, Shapiro RL, Zinner J, et al: The borderline ego and the working alliance: indications for family and individual treatment in adolescence. Int J Psychoanal 58:77–87, 1977

Stanton AH, Schwartz MS: The Mental Hospital: A Study of Institutional Participation in Psychiatric Illness and Treatment. New York, Basic Books, 1954

Stern DN: The Interpersonal World of the Infant: A View From Psychoanalysis and Developmental Psychology. New York, Basic Books, 1985

Waldinger RJ, Frank AF: Clinicians' experiences in combining medication and psychotherapy in the treatment of borderline patients. Hosp Community Psychiatry 40:712–718, 1989

CHAPTER 9

Supervision and Consultation

S upervision or consultation can provide a veritable life raft in the midst of all the crosscurrents inherent in working with borderline patients. As discussed in earlier chapters, levels of ego functioning, defenses, and transference-countertransference involvement can be transformed precipitously in any given session. Object relations can flip-flop, with the patient and therapist taking turns being the victim, abuser, and rescuer. Hate and sadism can contribute to the patient's becoming "special" just as effectively as inordinate dependency needs. Reliance on primitive defenses such as splitting and projective identification will constantly challenge the therapist's clinical skills. The patient's efforts to neutralize the therapist's analytic work ego through boundary seductions call for constant vigilance. The shifting transference-countertransference interactions demand corresponding modifications in therapeutic response to address the patient's "growth needs" and to avoid inappropriate gratification of "libidinal demands." At times, the only means available to the therapist to maintain the clinical flexibility necessary will be through outside help. Although we speak primarily about supervision, which is distinct from the consultation used by more advanced therapists, both have in common the provision of external support so important to the treatment of borderline personality disorder.

A significant countertransference pull during any session is to interact with the patient at the level of projective identification. Under such circumstances, everything is "now." Intense feelings are absolute. Self and other are reduced to fragmented parts. Abstracting abilities are concretized, and annihilation anxiety is rampant.

Given the pressure to communicate with the patient through unconscious, affectively laden roles in the patient's internal cast of characters, therapists may become hobbled in their efforts to sort through all the necessary diagnostic and clinical considerations. In short, the forest cannot be seen for the trees.

When communication between patient and therapist is dominated by projective identification, the crises associated with objects populating the patient's internal world become the only focus. Successful treatment requires a shift away from a communicative mode that is affectively driven and largely unconscious. Projective identification needs to be replaced by a capacity for both the patient and the therapist to participate in an analytic space (Ogden 1989). In this mode, both parties have the opportunity to reflect on the patient's desires and to "play" with their implications for the patient's relationships to actual, external objects. As Ogden wrote, the patient's individual psychological space recedes in importance during the treatment as the analytic experience between the patient and the clinician grows. Eventually, the analytic space existing between the two constitutes the therapeutic stage on which the patient's internal drama is experienced. With borderline patients, an analytic space is inordinately difficult to achieve and maintain.

When the therapist is mired in an unconscious, affectively dominated mode of communication, the restoration of analytic space is greatly needed. Supervision provides one avenue; the therapist's own psychotherapy provides another. The first focuses on understanding the patient better, and the second focuses on the therapist's self-understanding. We wish to emphasize that the unconscious projective identifications evoked in the therapist during the clinical process do not disappear in the supervisory process. Analytic space is not free of unconscious exchanges. In fact, during supervisory sessions, discovering the therapist's unconscious reactions to the patient can provide fertile diagnostic and clinical information. The affective intensity of the exchange with the patient is likely to get toned down, however, as the therapist reports to the supervisor what occurs in the therapy hour. A more cognitively dominated capacity for analytic space has the chance to emerge.

Both the therapist and the supervisor have a greater freedom than occurs within the therapy session to play with the ideas and reactions evoked by the patient's behavior.

As we hope to elaborate, the analytic space fostered by the supervision, and subsequently translated into work with the patient, is also informed by the presence and action of countertransference. Therapists working with analytic space allows themselves "to be created/molded by [their] patient in reality as well as in phantasy" (Ogden 1989, p. 89). In an analogous vein, supervisors must allow themselves to be created or molded by the clinical observations brought by the therapist as well as by the projective identifications enacted by the therapist. As a result, supervisors experience themselves in a manner that is specific to this therapist and this patient at this time. By examining personal psychological responses with the therapist, the supervisor can help untangle countertransference impasses and technical problems. Ultimately, the patient benefits.

The Therapist
Is Not Alone

Therapists treating patients with borderline personality disorder risk feeling isolated and all alone with the tormented inner world of their patients. The isolation to which we are referring takes on special qualities with these patients. Specifically, the patient's reliance on projective identification mandates that therapists partially surrender their personal sense of identity in the clinical crucible. The resulting "process identity" allows for greater reception and registration of the patient's transference but with the accompanying loss of certain aspects of the therapist's sense of self (Bollas 1983). To treat these individuals effectively, the therapist cannot expect otherwise. Thus, although the therapist's clinically observing ego may anticipate demands for fusion and nontherapeutic gratification, that awareness may do little to avert transference-countertransference enactment (Hirsch 1987).

The emergence of a process identity, together with its potential for an obliteration of the therapist's professional identity, can be conceptualized as the therapist's joining in a projective identification mode of communication. The therapist is coerced into experiencing aspects of the patient's internal world rather than having the opportunity to reflect on those aspects. Packed into the therapist's experience, or process identity, is the patient's sense of urgency, persecution, annihilation anxiety, affective volatility, and timelessness. When the patient leaves the session, more often than not, those feelings persist uncomfortably in the therapist. Rosenfeld's (1987) evocative description of "lavoratoric transference" amply captures the therapist's struggle to process the vestiges of the powerful projective identifications fostered by borderline patients. One of the most important capacities to recover in the wake of the session is the ability to think one's own thoughts about the coerced experience. Supervision can be invaluable in the therapist's reclaiming an analytic space from which to enrich the experiential knowledge of the patient gained through projective identification.

The question becomes how best to help the therapist reestablish an analytic space in the face of ubiquitous projective identification pressures. Traditional forms of supervision using retrospective examination of the session can fall short. An intellectual grasp may be achieved, but not necessarily an experiential grasp. Consequently, the therapist is left with chunks of unintegrated, raw affect. At best, retrospective consultation may help the therapist master a moment that has passed. But it does not address the introjected aspects of the patient that are currently alive in the therapist. Nor does it identify what exists in either the therapist or the patient that potentially can be triggered. Without attention to such experiential potentialities, therapists face the increasing probability that they will feel isolated and all alone in the tormented world of the borderline patient.

The therapist's risk of loneliness may be diminished by using the supervision to anticipate and analyze forthcoming sessions. Of course, neither the therapist nor the supervisor will be able to gaze into a crystal ball to know with certainty where the clinical process will lead. However, when the therapist's experience is dominated by chaos, the supervisor can provide stability through establishing reference points for future interventions. For example, the signal function of countertransference can be established to help the therapist diagnose the patient's internal state, practice silent interpretations, and employ self-analytic techniques. Countertransference tendencies to foreclose prematurely on an unfolding self-object relational paradigm or to enforce optimal distance rigidly can be anticipated and avoided. Powerful affects can be contained. As the therapist discovers that the experiential knowledge evoked through projective identifications can coexist with, and be complemented by, the enhancement of analytic space in the supervision, a new way of being with the patient can emerge.

What are the factors in the patient and in the therapist's countertransference that necessitate anticipatory exploration and external support? In the patient, the level of psychopathology, particularly with regard to aggressive conflicts that contribute to the patient's need to suffer, to destroy the treatment, and ultimately to descend into an intolerable sense of despair, is an important consideration. The strain on the therapists trying to empathize with a patient whose internal world is a violent and terrifying kaleidoscope is enormous (Carsky 1985–1986; Kernberg 1975; Searles 1967/1979). Outside help permits the therapist to sustain a treatment model in which interpretation of the patient's internal conflicts remains possible (Carsky 1985–1986).

The fragmentary countertransference intrinsic to working with borderline patients begs for the counterweight of an integrative learning experience available through supervision. Therapists pay a heavy toll when they constantly feel controlled, bullied, or badgered into playing a given role vis-à-vis the patient. The supervisor can protect the therapist's desire to help in the midst of siege by giving the therapist a respite, as well as a positive learning experience within the larger context of the patient's treatment. By functioning as a historian of the clinical process, the supervisor acts as an anchor when the therapist is buffeted about by the moment-to-moment demands of the patient. The sense of continuity and future orientation can offset the therapist's experience of frozen isolation.

Countertransference Awareness and Affect Tolerance

The task of supervision extends far beyond offering the therapist support when working with a particularly difficult patient. The therapist has come for supervision to learn how to be a better therapist. Toward that end, the supervisor must help the therapist tease apart and master many complex skills. With borderline patients, the lesson needs to be tailored in a particular way. Stated simply, a primary goal of supervision is to increase the therapist's ability to respond thoughtfully rather than to react reflexively. One means of enhancing the therapist's capacity for thoughtful intervention is to identify the signal function of countertransference (Friedman 1975).

To achieve this objective, the therapist must first become acquainted with the utility of countertransference awareness. Countertransference must be distinguished from clinical incompetence. A whole new clinical vista (particularly with the beginning therapist who is prone to attribute countertransference to personal experiences) is opened when the supervisor clarifies that these reactions are also reflective of the patient's internal functioning (Hunt 1981). Given this vantage, countertransference can be seen as fueling curiosity about how the therapist's reactions reflect the patient's needs and affect the therapy (Goin and Kline 1976). Examples for teaching the signal function of countertransference abound. The otherwise competent therapist's self-recriminations for being ineffective may stem from the patient's refusal to get better (Hamburg and Herzog 1990). Unwelcome erotic arousal may be stimulated by erotized demands to meet dependency needs. Hateful wishes can be elicited by the patient's underlying rage. Murderous thoughts can reflect the unconscious counterpart to the patient's overtly stated suicidal wishes. In each scenario, the signal function of countertransference can be used to understand the patient further once the therapist's internal conflicts are separated from feelings provoked by the patient.

The therapist must conceptualize the utility of countertransference awareness, as well as legitimize the powerful affects that are stirred. If the therapist cannot tolerate the strong negative and positive feelings evoked (whether erotic, loving, hateful, triumphant, or dependent), the theoretical advantage of countertransference awareness is nullified. This synthesis of affective tolerance and theoretical understanding is particularly germane to the treatment of borderline patients. Their porous boundaries and potential for misidentifying aspects of themselves as residing in the therapist can result in an uncanny and disturbing experience of countertransference fusion. Without some means of tolerating the intense affects the patient has deposited, the therapist may be compelled to act. Saying the right thing to the patient to avoid an imagined disaster then looms larger than understanding what the patient is trying to signal about inner thoughts and feelings.

Learning Alliance Between Therapist and Supervisor

When the therapist reveals intense countertransference affects to the supervisor, an intimate relationship is being forged between the two. Ideally, the learning alliance evolving between them is based on mutuality, respect, and collegiality (Book 1987). However, as with its clinical counterpart, the working alliance, the learning alliance is subject to resistances that derive from conflictual elements in both the therapist's and the supervisor's personalities (Doehrman 1976; Fleming and Benedek 1983). Although the therapist's emotional conflicts can be, and are, activated by the supervisory process, problems in the learning alliance need not be narrowly defined as pathological obstacles to be eliminated. Rather, to the extent learning difficulties represent the therapist's introjection of the patient's internal object relations, their exploration can catapult the therapist into a new realm of clinical mastery.

A long-standing debate exists over whether or not the intimate relationship between the therapist and the supervisor should be incorporated into the supervision (Ekstein and Wallerstein 1958; Fleming and Benedek 1983; Tarachow 1963). The supervisory process is easily compared with the clinical process with the patient. But are the two the same? Should the supervisor take a position akin to a clinician with the therapist and explore the nature and extent of the countertransference? Or is the learning alliance better served by a strictly didactic approach?

Valuable arguments are put forth by both sides. However, as Goin and Kline (1976) pointed out, the didactic, patient-centered approach is not so easily distinguished from the countertransference-informed, therapist-centered approach. For example, a supervisor who avoids discussion of the therapist's countertransference in an effort to protect the didactic process is behaving more like a clinician than an educator. The supervisor's caution is based on a fear that the budding transference might be stifled through premature interpretation. An educator would be less inhibited (Goin and Kline 1976). Conversely, if the supervisor points out how the therapist's identification with the patient constricts interventions, the intent is more didactic than clinical. The supervisor is concerned with bringing into the therapist's awareness what has been dissociated in the latter's clinical work with the patient (Issacharoff 1982).

From our point of view, neither approach is adequate in and of itself. Exclusive analysis of the countertransference in search of the patient can inappropriately emphasize the therapist's subjective experience over that of the patient's. Not only does the patient get lost, but the therapist may become increasingly defensive and confused with both the patient and the supervisor (Searles 1955/1965). In an exclusively didactic approach, supervisors who emphasize purely cognitive aspects place themselves outside the ongoing process existing between the therapist and the patient. As a result, the focus inevitably falls on the therapist's "inability" to treat the patent or "negative attitude" toward learning in supervision (Caligor 1981).

The process-oriented approach, which we advocate, requires that attention be paid to the interactions occurring between the patient and the therapist, as well as between the therapist and the supervisor. The learning difficulties manifested by the therapist in the supervision may stem from parallel difficulties encountered by the therapist in the work with the patient. Thus, Ekstein and Wallerstein (1958) noted, "even the rational questions of the [therapist], for which a mere didactic answer may suffice, are often based on specific affective problems the [therapist] has in both processes" (p. 178). Consequently, resolution of an existing tension between the therapist and the supervisor can often free the therapist to examine with greater spontaneity and competence the dynamics of the patient-therapist relationship (Doehrman 1976).

In working with borderline patients, the parallel tensions inevitably arising within the therapy and the supervision will be compounded by the influence of projective identification. To unearth the unconscious currents, both the therapist and the supervisor must actively participate in working with this particular patient at this particular time. The therapist actively engages with the patient through receiving and registering the process identity evoked by the patient's projective identifications. To a certain degree, the therapist, through internal monitoring, will be able to metabolize the fragments of primitive affect deposited by the patient. However, what the therapist's countertransference is signaling about the patient may be discovered only through the manifestation of that countertransference in the supervisory relationship.

The supervisor actively participates in the treatment of the patient by helping the therapist identify the process identity that the patient has evoked in the therapist. Toward this end, the supervisor must allow perceptions of the patient to be shaped by clinical observations brought by the therapist as well as the unconscious projective identifications presented by the therapist. Although the "inside" experience of the supervisor will be qualitatively different from that of the therapist, each will be struggling through the patient's material.

Interchangeability of the Evoker and Recipient Roles

We spoke in earlier chapters about how the transference-countertransference paradigm is jointly created between the patient and the therapist. In a parallel fashion, the therapist and the supervisor can examine the therapeutic process through a jointly created crucible in which aspects of their relationship may be understood as reflecting the patient's internal world. Although tracking parallel processes is valuable in any supervisory situation, the ability of the therapist and the supervisor to switch roles and play the evoker or the recipient is particularly helpful in the work with borderline patients. For example, therapists are recipients of the urgent, raw affects evoked by the patient. Therapists may not consciously be able to acknowledge their impact of those affects that resonate with their own repressed or split-off aspects. When therapists then arrive for supervision, they become evokers of such experiences with the supervisor. In turn, as Caligor (1981) observed, the supervisor as recipient can become the evoker within a peer supervisory group.

By comparing and contrasting the interchangeable evoker and recipient roles, the therapist and the supervisor have the opportunity experientially to sample and cognitively to examine various aspects of the patient's transference. For example, the supervisor may identify an uncharacteristic feeling of irritability or impotence with the therapist during a supervisory session. Together they can explore the possibility that the supervisor's unusual reaction is evidence of a projective identification enactment. Through discussion or role playing, the supervisor can help the therapist lay claim to the irritability and impotence embedded in the negative countertransference. The supervisor, as recipient of unwanted negative countertransference, evokes such feelings once again in the therapist while facilitating conscious integration of the patient's impact on the therapist. Other chances for integration arise when the therapist identifies with one part of the patient's inner thoughts and feelings and the supervisor another. Although reasons for divergent perceptions of the patient may be numerous, the therapist and the supervisor can evaluate the possibility that they are responding differentially to the patient's split-off good and bad self-representations. The kinds of splitting problems described in Chapter 8 may also occur in supervision.

Searles (1955/1965) cautioned that situations may arise in which the therapist's, or even the supervisor's, anxiety may be more intense than that of either of the other two participants. Therapists may be projecting similar aspects of their personal experience onto both the supervisor and the patient. Since such projections cause therapists to behave in a comparable manner toward each of the other two parties, supervisors should be able to observe similarities between the therapists' modes of functioning in the supervisory relationship and their modes of functioning in the therapeutic relationship (Searles 1955/1965). In such instances, the roles of evoker and recipient are not interchangeable, and the treatment process is stuck.

Supervisors also may be projecting aspects of their own emotional conflict into both the therapist and the patient. When this occurs, supervisors perceive the therapist and the patient as strikingly similar in their modes of operation. Teitelbaum (1990) termed the supervisor's blind spot *supertransference*. Whether the supertransference stems from reactivated inner conflicts, specific reactions to the individual therapist, or countertransference reactions to the therapist's transference, constriction of the supervisor's teaching capacity needs to be self-monitored (Teitelbaum 1990).

What may look like an invitation by the therapist for the supervisor to enact a supertransference may actually be an important opportunity to get to know the patient. For example, the illusion may exist in the therapist's mind that the supervisor "knows best" or is "objective." The therapist's wish for the supervisor to treat the patient for the therapist could tempt the supervisor to become the omnipotent rescuer. Rather than accepting the role of "knowing best," the supervisor's task more appropriately becomes one of helping the therapist identify the rescue wish received from the patient and evoked in the supervisor.

Narrow Versus Broad
Countertransference

From our perspective, countertransference is examined in the supervisory relationship only so far as it assists in the therapist's learning self-analysis and in no way violates the therapist's privacy (Hunt 1981). With the supervisor's encouragement, the therapist may reveal feelings about the patient and clarify the relevant interactions, insights about personal experiences, or work with other patients (Rinsley 1989). Because such bits of self-analysis assist in a constructive process of integrating and working through a piece of learning, the supervisor can be most helpful by being an accepting audience and nothing more (Hunt 1981). The therapist's emotional reactions are used as a starting point through which the patient can be better known. The predominant focus is on the here-and-now aspects of the therapist's reactions. In personal analysis or psychotherapy, emotional reactions can be explored in depth and used as a departure point through which the therapists can know themselves better (Hunt 1981).

The integration and working through of a piece of learning draws on elements of both narrow and broad countertransference. Stated differently, therapists are challenged to broaden their self-awareness to include an appreciation of the patient's influence as distinct from their own personal perceptions. Likewise, therapists are challenged to narrow the depth of their emotional involvement to the degree that their appropriate desire to help the patient becomes distinct from other self-serving needs. The therapist's pivotal, integrative role in the therapy process is highlighted when we consider that self-awareness is usually least in the patient and greatest in the supervisor, and the depth of emotional involvement is usually greatest in the patient and least in the supervisor (Searles 1955/1965).

The interplay of narrow and broad variants of countertransference is illustrated in the following vignette:

In contrast to her dark mood in the previous few sessions, Ms. G began this appointment euphorically describing her passion for dancing. Her exuberance disappeared suddenly with the dour observation that she needed more intensive treatment. In fact, she needed the freedom to telephone Dr. Q, her therapist, at the slightest hint of distress. The therapist believed firmly that such frequent, boundariless contact would invite regression. Yet sheepishly, she thought about her own apparent limitations in treating this woman. After all, the patient's progress had been very slow. Privately, Dr. Q wished that she were more skilled. She had frequently discussed this dilemma in supervision. How should she respond to the patient's inordinate demands, particularly when she felt so inadequate in treating her? Propped up by her supervisor's advice on what to say, she told the patient that she was quite interested in learning what would help her treatment be more intensive. "Intensive," she clarified, meant a deepening of therapeutic process, and not the addition of numerous phone calls. Ms. G agreed that unlimited use of the phone was not a solution to her distress and said that she wanted to talk further about making the therapy more intensive.

That night Dr. Q had an extremely unsettling dream. She awoke anxiously with the concern that her body was being controlled from within by an alien force. Her immediate association was to Ms. G. She had absolutely no doubt that the alien force she had experienced represented her patient's control of her. Distressed and angered that Ms. G had such influence over her internal life, Dr. Q had difficulty going back to sleep.

Two days after the dream, the patient began her session by asserting how alive she felt when having sex or dancing. Ms. G described orgasmic sensations that she experienced at various points in her early childhood, which she felt her mother abhorred. Dr. Q commented about the patient's mother's taking away her pleasure. Without skipping a beat, Ms. G added that her mother had taken away her dancing too.

Ms. G's erotized and hypomanic stance suddenly shifted. She became extremely devaluing of the therapist and demanded to phone her whenever she felt stressed. Therapy could help Ms. G only if she knew that she had access to the therapist! She lamented that the treatment was making her worse! She went on to say, "Besides, you promised me your home phone number last session! I told you about the warmth and comfort I felt when I have sex or dance only because I believed your promise!"

With accusations of betrayal, the patient railed against Dr. Q's attempts to clarify that making the treatment more "intensive" did not mean unlimited phone access. Ms. G ended the session angrily saying that Dr. Q was trying to drive her crazy. The therapist felt dismayed. Ms. G was not the only one who felt like she was being driven crazy.

As if she were on a mission to bargain down the price with a used car salesperson, the patient began the next session calmly stating that she would talk of nothing else until they had a plan for phone contact. If Dr. Q would not let Ms. G call her directly, could she at least instruct her answering service to put the patient directly through to her? She had to know the plan. Convincing herself that the therapist would not budge, Ms. G complained of the therapist's lack of integrity, then she begged for Dr. Q to specify what she had to do to get Dr. Q to change her mind. She hinted that she would become suicidal.

Somewhat off balance, Dr. Q tried to explain that when her back was against the wall, they had no room to talk with each other. She tried to empathize with Ms. G's desperation and encouraged her to say more about her sense of urgency. Ms. G countered by saying that being able to phone her doctor was imperative for the success of her treatment. She absolutely refused to talk about her urgency, saying, "So you won't let me call you when I'm in crisis! You just want me to talk about what's going on with me. I won't do that! I won't tell you! There are all kinds of things that I need to talk to you about—but what's the use!?"

The following session was more of the same. Utterly frustrated, Dr. Q could feel herself losing her resolve. She did not want Ms. G to become too upset because she feared that the patient would become suicidal. Gratification seemed to be the only way to avert a suicidal regression, as well as to stop Ms. G's lacerating devaluation. She was aware that her discomfort was hobbling her therapeutic effectiveness and distorting her assessment of the patient. She hated herself for having lost so much control. She hated the patient for ripping apart everything that she tried to offer her. Her dream of being manipulated by an alien force returned to her mind, and she hated the patient's invasion into her private life.

About two-thirds of the way through the session, Ms. G announced, "I won't see you any more!" Additionally, she enumerated her primary relationships and vowed to cut off each one. Dr. Q felt desperate. The patient explained that her actions would hurt her more than they hurt the therapist and walked out of the room supposedly never to return.

Exasperated, Dr. Q thought about what had just happened. She was happy that Ms. G had left. Good riddance! But, despite her best efforts, her nagging and reluctant worry about what Ms. G might do next would not be assuaged. She walked out past her waiting room to the street and found Ms. G sobbing by the front door.

Dr. Q told Ms. G that she was greatly concerned about her walking out on her treatment. Tearfully, the patient indicated that her exit had hurt her terribly. When they returned to the office, to the therapist's relief, Ms. G was quite docile. Within minutes, however, she was angrily demanding to have Dr. Q's phone number. Finally, as a compromise, Ms. G offered to present a written request at the end of each session for phone access to the therapist. That way, Dr. Q would not forget her "need," and they could spend their time talking about her "real" problems. Thinking this absurd, Dr. Q told her that they needed to talk rather than pass notes. The patient, now exasperated, ended the session with bitter complaints.

Dr. Q could not wait to get to the sanctuary of her supervisor's office. Although initially inhibited by her guilt, she began to describe her exasperation. The dream about the controlling alien force became a springboard for revealing how much she hated Ms. G. The more she talked, the more the therapist was surprised by the intensity of her feelings. Dr. R, the supervisor, agreed that he felt some of the same feelings, although to a lesser degree, in hearing about the interactions with the patient. The experience of working with this patient at this time became increasingly palpable to the supervisor.

Feeling guilty, ashamed, and optionless, Dr. Q became shaky all over. She had difficulty concentrating on Dr. R's advice. The supervisor also felt somewhat helpless because his words were not freeing the therapist from the patient's alien grasp. Dr. R had become the recipient, in a toned-down fashion, of the therapist's exasperation. Through observing this uncharacteristic interaction between themselves, the therapist and supervisor were able to discuss the patient's alien presence within the supervisory hour. Together, they were able to identify the therapist's counteridentification to the patient's greed and envy. Her sense of inadequacy stemmed from the impossible task of trying to satisfy this woman. Her efforts fell short of Ms. G's expectations, and as a result, Ms. G applied increasing pressure. Her hate sprang, in part, from Ms. G's tormenting, unrealistic demands. Now able to understand Dr. R's suggested interventions in an intellectual fashion, Dr. Q remained emotionally skeptical.

When Dr. R asked his supervisee if she could behave differently in her role vis-à-vis the patient, Dr. Q honestly observed, "Not yet." She asked the supervisor to keep talking with her to help her further untangle herself from the "alien" introject. Dr. R assured her that she had several days before she met with the patient again and that she did not have to digest the suggested interventions or choose at that moment what she wanted to do. She should not expect the choking alien presence to disappear simply because she had confessed to it in supervision. Rather than discuss specific things that the therapist could say to the patient, they focused on the therapist's experience of being controlled and tormented. The supervisor said that he, too, felt hindered because of the patient's crippling effect on the therapist, and he pointed out how their learning alliance had been disrupted. In contrast to an earlier phase of treatment when Ms. G was severely regressed and they had focused on the importance of the patient's survival, now the therapist and supervisor spoke of the importance of the *therapist's* survival. They agreed on the therapeutic value of telling the patient that she could not torment the therapist any more.

Dr. Q tried to prepare herself to make such an intervention by forecasting the patient's reaction. She described her fantasy of the patient's acting mortally wounded by the intrusion of the therapist's appraisal of reality. She spoke about her consciously preferred strategy of not doing anything to disappoint Ms. G. Then Dr. Q laughed at herself because she seemed to be saying that she would rather have the patient invade her dreams than to become the patient's worst nightmare! With this discovery of her unconscious entanglement with the patient, Dr. Q was prepared to engage in a more routine collaboration with her supervisor. She had broken through to an analytic space.

She confessed her exasperation at the patient's proposal that she present her with a note each session requesting frequent phone contact. When asked what caused the therapist to refuse Ms. G's offer, Dr. Q explained that she considered her job to be one of getting the patient to use her ego—to put her thoughts and feelings into words rather than concretize them in a note. Dr. R observed that he would have immediately taken the patient up on her offer. He explained that if the patient could stick to her promise to talk about her "real" problems, then the note writing served an ego function, albeit contrived. If she could not stick to her promise, then the therapist could confront her ongoing disruption of a productive therapeutic relationship. Here the therapist learned something that her countertransference had prevented her from understanding before.

Finally, they spoke of a treatment strategy in which the best defense was a good offense. The therapist was encouraged to start the meeting by telling the patient that she did not want to be tormented any more with requests to have unlimited phone access. Dr. Q could tell Ms. G that she would accept her notes, and they could then move on to discuss more substantive issues. The supervisor explained that by taking the initiative, Dr. Q would startle the patient and secure her therapeutic footing. This strategy was preferable to having Ms. G's scathing complaints preemptively knock the therapist off balance. Dr. Q was relieved to have the supervisor's encouragement to reestablish herself as a clinician and thankful to be able to shed her role as the repository for the patient's greed and envy.

Supervisor as a Container

The foregoing vignette illustrates the importance of the containing function in supervision. The identification of Dr. R's intense affective reaction through the therapist's report, the supervisor's resonance, and the uncharacteristic disruption of their learning alliance served to rein in the fragmenting emotional impact of the patient's projective identifications. Recall how the exasperation felt by Dr. Q bounded back and forth between her and Ms. G. To a much lesser degree, Dr. R noted that he felt helpless when the formulations he offered to Dr. Q did not settle her into her normal learning routine. Instead, she was distracted by hateful, tormented, exasperated, and guilty feelings. The alien entanglement interfering with her clinical competence could shift only when those affects were no longer so urgent. By helping the therapist to translate her feelings into words, the supervisor provided containment and paved the way for transformation of the parallel experience bouncing back and forth among the patient, therapist, and supervisor.

Affective containment is enhanced by the greater freedom to speak in the supervisory setting about feelings available to the therapist and the supervisor. For example, Dr. Q's revelation to Dr. R of feeling controlled by an alien force was something that he would not have said to the patient. The supervisor, in turn, can be much more self-disclosing about fantasies and emotions evoked by the therapist's reports and the patient's behavior than would be possible in the patient's presence. Burke's (1992) suggestion that hearing about the therapist's feelings in psychotherapy may diminish the patient's affective intensity seems to have a parallel in supervision when the therapist hears about the supervisor's feelings. After Dr. R revealed that he, too, felt crippled by the patient's impact, Dr. Q was able to unearth her fear of becoming the patient's worst nightmare. The result was a greater freedom to be explicit about the affective discourse. At the same time, clinical theory could be introduced to translate further affects into words and concepts.

Part of the challenge before the supervisor is to help the therapist disentangle from the fragmented countertransference. In Chapter 2 we spoke of the importance of the therapist's supporting the patient's "growth needs" based on the patient's need for ego support. In contrast, "libidinal demands" stemming from the patient's conflicts are best left ungratified. Every supervisory session embodies a comparable dilemma of how to manage the countertransference being identified. The patient's "libidinal needs" can be equated roughly with the therapist's narrow countertransference. The patient's "growth needs" can be compared roughly with the therapist's broad countertransference. Although a parallel exists, management of countertransference in supervision is not identical to the management of the clinical process in psychotherapy. First, the personally rooted, narrow countertransference is best dealt with in the therapist's own treatment outside the supervision. With regard to the therapist's broad countertransference, or growth needs, the task of supervision is specific. Assistance is needed to integrate an identity as a therapist in the face of the patient's unidimensional and coercive transference demands.

For example, identifying the therapist's tormented process identity was an important part of Dr. Q's supervision. This information was absolutely necessary for the containment of what the patient had evoked. The supervisor could assist the therapist in translating the alien, visceral experience of Ms. G, once it was consciously acknowledged and contained, into a more abstract, conceptual mode of understanding her needs and intentions. By identifying how the fragmented process identities intrinsic to working with Ms. G at that particular time dovetail, Dr. Q could reclaim an integrated sense of herself as a therapist distinct from the circumscribed role of evoker or recipient. This integration of therapeutic identity was dramatically illustrated by Dr. Q's initial confusion and inability to concentrate on what Dr. R was saying. She felt that supervision was not helping at all. As her unconscious entanglement became clearer to her, she regained her identity as a functional therapist. She was prepared to return to the therapy process in a therapeutic role. Given this perspective, countertransference can be understood not only as information coming from the patient, but also the containment and working through of countertransference can be seen as returning information back to the patient. After the containing function of supervision helped Dr. Q get back on track, the next session with Ms. G was strikingly different.

> At the beginning of the hour, Dr. Q initiated the conversation. She said that Ms. G's repeated requests for unlimited phone contact caused them to go around in tormenting and pointless circles. She stated frankly that she was not willing to be tormented any more. Further, she assumed that the repetition was tormenting to Ms. G, too. She accepted Ms. G's suggestion of writing a note so that they could talk about other important things in her life. Finally, Dr. Q reminded Ms. G that when they had come close to such a discussion before, Ms. G responded by fleeing the session. Dr. Q stated that if the patient needed to leave, she would respect Ms. G's decision. She would be there when Ms. G was ready to come back.
>
> First appearing confused, then surprised, then callously rejected, Ms. G quickly blurted out, "If I want to leave, you're going to let me! Just like that? You're telling me to leave!! I can't believe it! I'm quitting therapy!" Dr. Q responded calmly. She clarified that she was not directing the patient to leave, simply explaining that she would be fine if Ms. G went away and would also be there when she returned. The patient leaped from her chair and announced her intention to walk out. The therapist was dismayed and less comfortable than she had hoped with the idea of being left alone with

her thoughts about this woman. However, she said calmly, "I'm not planning on going anywhere. I'll be here when you get back."

Ms. G produced an impressive display of guilt-inducing pyrotechnics. But Dr. Q stood firm. She noted privately that in contrast to the previous few sessions, she felt detached and unimpressed. She wondered if she was unconsciously isolating affect or if she simply was in the role of an adult who was not impressed with a 2-year-old's temper tantrum.

Abruptly, and without the emotional intensity displayed moments before, Ms. G said, "You've changed!" Her statement felt like both an indictment of betrayal and a simple observation of fact to the therapist. Apparently alarmed at Dr. Q's newfound ability to exist outside her control, Ms. G brought out the artillery. She blasted Dr. Q for her callous disregard for her needs. She compared the therapist unfavorably with several important people in her life. In particular, she compared Dr. Q with a highly idealized professor who previously had taken her under her wing. The professor would have known how to help her because she was brilliant! She would not let her go!

Dr. Q felt pulled to defend herself. She slipped in the direction of reassuring the patient that she would never leave her (or disappoint her) by reminding her that she had gone to look for her when Ms. G left the office the week before. However, silently taking inventory of her feelings, the therapist noticed that she wanted to prevent the patient from leaving again and that she wanted to dazzle the patient with her intellect like the professor. With this self-observation, the therapist managed to avoid further countertransference enactment.

In the next instant Ms. G ventured onto new ground by asking herself if the professor's presence would, in fact, make her better. Dr. Q quickly reinforced her psychological thinking by saying, "These are very important questions. By asking them, you give yourself space, and you give us space, to do the work of therapy. Such space becomes available by asking questions rather than making tormenting demands for action." Ms. G's response was to ask once again for phone-calling privileges. Dr. Q felt pulled in, sorry, guilty. She wanted to rescue the patient from her pain. Ms. G kept demanding an "explanation" for why she was feeling so badly. She tried to shame the therapist by saying the professor would explain to her the genetic roots of her distress. Dr. Q decided to "explain" by making a simple observation about the process unfolding between them. She said, "I think you're trying to push me away with your words."

The patient paused, then regrouped for the next onslaught. She reminded the therapist more and more of a 2 year old having a dramatic temper tantrum. Under the circumstances, Dr. Q decided that her best response would be to sit by and wait. In her own time, Ms. G returned to an analytic space. However, first, she had to complain about the therapist's letting her down. Then she focused for some minutes on her disappointment in her mother, who had caused all of her current problems. Slowly, she became more thoughtful and observed that she had always been fond of her mother. Her assertion that her mother was an absolute monster did not fit with her recollection of warm moments. Maybe her mother was not so distant after all. Finally, she asked herself and Dr. Q if it were possible that she had pushed her mother away. Maybe her mother was not so bad. Maybe she just couldn't accept what her mother had to offer.

Once again Dr. Q reinforced Ms. G's psychological thinking by noting that such questions allowed them to explore the tough weekends, social isolation, and bad dreams to which she often alluded. Her demands for unlimited phone contact prevented any such discussion. Reflectively, Ms. G wondered what made it so hard for her to engage in such discussions. Before she could answer her own question, she returned to her pyrotechnic display, insisting bitterly that the therapist did not understand how much she suffered. She angrily accused Dr. Q once again, saying, "You've changed!" In response to the accusation, Dr. Q repeated calmly, "I think you're trying to push me away with your words. I'm not planning on going anywhere."

Although Dr. Q's comment captured exactly what was happening between them, it did not "explain" the specific content to the patient's satisfaction. Even so, while she continued to complain, she also settled down a bit. She watched the clock, and with 2 minutes left, she begged Dr. Q not to leave her. Again, she said that she was not planning on disappearing. Ms. G left appearing relieved.

When Dr. Q described this session to her supervisor, Dr. R concurred with the patient. Dr. Q had changed. The therapist recalled that she had continued to feel shaky when she left supervision the week before. In fact, she had been frightened when she began the meeting with Ms. G. But she had resolved to say directly to the patient what she could and could not tolerate. She noted, "The more she acted like a 2 year old, the more resolved I felt to protect the therapy and not get caught up in attempting to gratify her demands. I was better able to observe the tugs in me to rescue her, to defend myself, to compete with the professor, to prevent her from leaving, and to resist succumbing to my hate." The therapist and her supervisor agreed that the supervision had been an important container through which Dr. Q had regained this therapeutic expertise and achieved a more integrated understanding of the patient.

Comparison of Supervision and Consultation

Supervision is generally reserved for the beginning or intermediate therapist who is striving to master the complex skills required in psychotherapy. Often the supervision takes place under the auspices of an academic or training program. Because of the therapist's training status, legal and ethical responsibility for the treatment of the patient rests on the supervisor's shoulders. Consequently, the therapist is expected to implement a treatment strategy that has been discussed in the supervisory process. As a result of the unavoidable authoritarian cast to the supervisory relationship, as well as the therapist's dependence on the supervisor for performance evaluations and recommendations, their work together is vulnerable to contamination by the therapist's superego projections (Doehrman 1976). The supervisor needs great sensitivity to help the therapist navigate this complex interpersonal field toward the goal of successful learning.

Consultation generally occurs when the advanced clinician seeks the opinion of a colleague regarding a particularly thorny problem. The consultant is asked to help the therapist tackle a focused clinical impasse on a time-limited basis. Superego projections are somewhat diminished by the collegial nature of the relationship. Although the consultant's expertise is highly valued, the advice given need not be implemented. Ultimate responsibility for the treatment of the patient rests with the therapist and not with the consultant.

Despite the reality of the consultant-consultee relationship, in many instances the therapist who seeks consultation may anticipate censure or disapproval. Therapists often feel ashamed that they cannot manage a difficult clinical situation on their own, and they fear that the consultant will regard them as incompetent. When erotic countertransference feelings are involved, the therapist may view the consultant as an even greater superego figure than the supervisor would be. As we noted in Chapter 6, some therapists, in the early stages of lovesickness, may feel that their own ethical standards are slipping. The fear that the consultant will react like a harsh conscience may also be a wish to have their own beleaguered superego bolstered by external sources. Indeed, one of the values of consultation is that therapists who have lost their bearings can have their sense of psychological equilibrium restored. Borderline patients make therapists doubt their own judgment. An uninvolved third party has the necessary objectivity to help the therapist see the clinical situation with greater clarity.

What supervision and consultation have in common, which is so important in the treatment of borderline patients, is the use of external support to manage countertransference. Identifying the precise composition of countertransference, whether narrow or broad, is quite complicated. Even an experienced therapist who has a sophisticated theoretical understanding of such constellations encounters difficulty in always responding professionally, unless assisted by consultation (Carsky 1985–1986). Although the need for education varies across different skill levels, the challenge to make sense of and respond to the countertransference evoked by this patient group remains constant. Education, on which beginning therapists are dependent, can be described as the acquisition of the art of utilizing knowledge (Issacharoff 1982). For our purposes, a fundamental element of knowledge required of all therapists in the treatment of borderline patients is the art of utilizing countertransference.

Summary

Many beginning therapists are reluctant to share intense countertransference feelings in supervision. Just as therapist and patient forge a therapeutic alliance, supervisor and supervisee must develop a learning alliance that allows for free expression of the beginning therapist's countertransference reactions. The optimal approach to supervision is to steer a middle course between an exclusive analysis of the countertransference and an exclusively didactic focus on cognitive aspects of the treatment. The process that occurs between supervisee and supervisor often reflects what is transpiring between therapist and patient. Feelings evoked in the therapist by the patient may also be evoked in the supervisor by the supervisee. When the therapist's primitive and raw affects are unmetabolized, the supervisor may be used as a container to help modify those affects. Although consultation generally occurs with less frequency and is used by more experienced clinicians, the same parallel processes observed in supervision may also apply to the consultative relationship.

References

Bollas C: Expressive uses of the countertransference: notes to the patient from oneself. Contemporary Psychoanalysis 19:1–34, 1983

Book HE: The resident's countertransference: approaching an avoided topic. Am J Psychother 41:555–562, 1987

Burke WF: Countertransference disclosure and the asymmetry/mutuality dilemma. Psychoanalytic Dialogues 2:241–271, 1992

Caligor L: Parallel and reciprocal processes in psychoanalytic supervision. Contemporary Psychoanalysis 17:1–27, 1981

Carsky M: The resolution in impasses in long-term intensive, inpatient psychotherapy. Int J Psychoanal 11:435–454, 1985–1986

Doehrman MJG: Parallel processes in supervision and in psychotherapy. Bull Menninger Clin 40:9–104, 1976

Ekstein R, Wallerstein RS: The Teaching and Learning Psychotherapy. New York, Basic Books, 1958

Fleming J, Benedek TF: Psychoanalytic Supervision: A Method of Clinical Teaching. New York, International Universities Press, 1983

Friedman HJ: Psychotherapy of borderline patients: the influence of theory on technique. Am J Psychiatry 1:1048–1052, 1975

Goin MK, Kline F: Countertransference: a neglected subject in clinical supervision. Am J Psychiatry 133(1):41–44, 1976

Hamburg P, Herzog D: Supervising the therapy of patients with eating disorders. Am J Psychother 44:369–380, 1990

Hirsch I: Varying modes of analytic participation. J Am Acad Psychoanal 15:205–222, 1987

Hunt W: The use of countertransference in psychotherapy supervision. J Am Acad Psychoanal 9:361–373, 1981

Issacharoff A: Countertransference in supervision: therapeutic consequences for the supervisee. Contemporary Psychoanalysis 18:455–472, 1982

Kernberg OF: Borderline Conditions and Pathological Narcissism. New York, Jason Aronson, 1975

Ogden TH: The Primitive Edge of Experience. Northvale, NJ, Jason Aronson, 1989

Rinsley DB: Developmental Pathogenesis and Psychoanalytic Treatment of Borderline and Narcissistic Personalities. Northvale, NJ, Jason Aronson, 1989

Rosenfeld H: Impasse and Interpretation: Therapeutic and Anti-Therapeutic Factors in the Psychoanalytic Treatment of Psychotic, Borderline, and Neurotic Patients. London, Tavistock, 1987

Searles HF: The informational value of the supervisor's emotional experiences (1955), in Collected Papers on Schizophrenia and Related Subjects. New York, International Universities Press, 1965, pp 157–176

Searles HF: The "dedicated physician" in the field of psychotherapy and psychoanalysis (1967), in Countertransference and Related Subjects. Madison, CT, International Universities Press, 1979, pp 71–88

Tarachow S: An Introduction to Psychotherapy. New York, International Universities Press, 1963

Teitelbaum SH: Supertransference: the role of the supervisor's blind spots. Psychoanalytic Psychology 7:243–258, 1990

CHAPTER 10

Therapeutic Aspects of Managing Countertransference

T he focus of this volume has been the management of counter-transference in the treatment of borderline patients. Success-ful psychotherapy clearly involves many other factors besides attention to countertransference. In therapies that are situated at the expressive end of the expressive-supportive continuum, tech-niques such as interpretation of transference, confrontation of splitting, and clarification of distortions may be essential. When therapists select more supportive strategies based on a careful psy-chodynamic assessment of the patient's strengths and weaknesses, they are likely to use interventions such as encouragement, advice, praise, reframing, education, direct and indirect strengthening of ego functions, and limit setting (Rockland 1992).

As we noted in Chapter 1, management of countertransference is nevertheless the foundation on which the rest of the treatment depends. Therapists who react to their fear of the patient's wrath by failing to set limits, or who respond to their feelings of rage at the patient by making interpretations tinged with hostility and sadism, are not functioning effectively. They may have mastered the tools of the trade, but the use of those tools has been contaminated and impaired by overpowering feelings.

More fundamentally, unmanaged countertransference may make forming a viable therapeutic alliance with the patient next to impossible. The patient's ability to collaborate with the therapist, based on the perception that the therapist is helpful and working toward commonly held goals, is essential for effective psychotherapy. Indeed, the therapeutic alliance has been cited as one of the principal vehicles for change in the psychotherapy of borderline patients (Gabbard et al. 1988; Horwitz 1974; Meissner 1988). Transference-countertransference enactments constantly threaten to disrupt the alliance in the treatment of borderline patients, because the perception of the therapist as helpful is fragile and easily undermined by the sensitive attunement of the patient to the therapist's every nuance.

Beyond the therapeutic alliance, the management of countertransference may be therapeutic in and of itself. Having said that a range of expressive and supportive interventions are instrumental to psychotherapy, we would also argue that the various methods of handling countertransference described in the foregoing chapters may be profoundly therapeutic and responsible, at least in part, for positive changes. Before considering the ways in which countertransference management is therapeutic, however, we should first review what is known about the mechanisms of change in psychotherapy in general.

Mechanisms of Change in Psychotherapy

Psychoanalysis and highly expressive psychodynamic psychotherapy rely heavily on the use of interpretation as the instrument of therapeutic change. Whether or not the therapeutic relationship itself is of equal importance in producing change is the subject of considerable controversy (Cooper 1988, 1992; Gabbard 1994; Hamilton 1988; Meissner 1991). The classical psychoanalytic view is that therapeutic action depends on intrapsychic conflict resolution brought about through accurate transference interpretations (Strachey 1934). The therapist or analyst interprets the patient's id impulses and wishes toward the therapist or analyst and the defenses against those wishes and impulses. After a period of working through, the patient comes to realize that the feelings are actually displaced from childhood figures to the therapist or analyst. The cognitive grasp of these interpretations allows for the taming of the superego and the expansion of the ego.

In recent years the influence of the object relations–interpersonal model of psychoanalysis has shifted the understanding of the therapeutic action to the effects of a new relationship with the analyst or therapist. Loewald (1960/1980) anticipated this shift when he compared analysis with a reparenting process in which the patient internalizes aspects of the analyst in the same way the child internalizes a parent. Ogden (1979, 1986, 1989) extended these ideas further in his conceptualization of projective identification as the transformation and return (in modified form) of the patient's projected contents. The holding function of the therapist or analyst and the reintrojection by the patient result in a change in the interactional mode between therapist and patient such that both of them generate a new way of experiencing old psychological contents.

Pulver (1992) and Cooper (1992) sought to integrate the role of insight and a new relationship in bringing about change. Pulver argued that the "either-or" polarization of insight through interpretation and alterations in the self through a new relationship is artificial. He stressed that "an understanding relationship cannot be maintained without insight into the dynamics of the relationship itself" (p. 204). From this perspective, he suggested that the two always must work in concert. Cooper stressed that the new interpersonal relationship in and of itself produces insight. It creates sufficient affective and cognitive dissonance that insight in the form of an alteration of one's internal self- and object-representations and their affective interaction is necessary to accommodate the internal pressures. He believed that the interpretation of content is less important than how the therapist and patient are relating to one another. Luborsky (1984) argued that, in the vast majority of psychotherapies, change occurs partly from interpretive mechanisms and partly from direct effects of the relationship.

In supportive psychotherapy the mechanisms of change depend explicitly on noninterpretive interventions and the relationship itself. Wallerstein's (1986) research stemming from the Menninger Foundation Psychotherapy Research Project delineated a number of mechanisms of change in supportive psychotherapy that led to lasting improvements at long-term follow-up. Although the Menninger project was begun at a time when borderline personality disorder was not a fashionable diagnosis, many of those patients would now be classified as borderline. One of these mechanisms was the transference cure effected through an unanalyzed positive, dependent transference. Another mechanism of change involved the acknowledgment of the patient's need to be a "therapeutic lifer" (pp. 690–691). In these cases the therapist recognized that the patient could not completely terminate and arranged for the patient to have infrequent contacts—anywhere from once a month to once every 6 months. These patients could sustain a high level of functioning as long as they knew the contact with the therapist would continue indefinitely.

Wallerstein (1986) also described a phenomenon he termed "transfer of the transference" (p. 692) as another supportive mechanism of cure. In these cases the positive dependency on the therapist was transferred to another person, usually, but not always, a spouse. Certain patients seemed to change by defying the therapist, and Wallerstein referred to these as "the antitransference cure" (p. 693). Still other cases in the Menninger sample seemed to change through a narrowly defined variant of the corrective emotional experience in which the patient's transference behavior was met by the therapist with steady concern and neutrality. Finally, direct, nonjudgmental advice was important in effecting change in other patients. Wallerstein described this process as "reality testing and re-education" (p. 694).

Rockland (1992), who wrote extensively about psychodynamically oriented supportive therapy for borderline patients, described several categories of therapeutic action, some of which are similar to Wallerstein's (1986). In addition, he noted that the systematic strengthening of the patient's ego functions may produce lasting change. He also described positive feedback loops that involve interactions with significant others outside treatment. Patients who become less paranoid, for example, because of positive interactions with a therapist will find that other people begin responding in more supportive and trusting ways. These interactions allow the patients to become even less paranoid, and so forth, until the change is durable.

Countertransference and the Management of the Relationship

In light of the broad consensus that the new relationship offered by the therapist to the patient is central to the healing effects of both expressive and supportive psychotherapy, management of counter-transference is therapeutic principally because it is the primary de-terminant of how the therapeutic relationship is presented to the patient. Therapists who *react* to the patient's projective identifica-tion by becoming a present-day version of an object from the past merely confirm the patient's internal world and close off the oppor-tunity for new experience. On the other hand, the therapist who holds, contains, and *responds* to the patient cleanses and detoxifies the projected distortions and presents a modified version of the object for reintrojection (along with a new mode of object related-ness). This projective-introjective sequence is the essence of the psy-chotherapeutic process (Scharff 1992). Just as the mother modifies infantile preconceptions through her containment of the infant's projective identifications, the therapist alters the internal world of the patient through containment. Mental representations always maintain some connection with the original internal objects, but containment makes possible the acquisition of increasing auton-omy from the archaic objects (Ogden 1986).

As we have stressed in the preceding chapters, successful han-dling of the patient's projections involves experiencing the full force of them without being completely taken over by them to the point that the therapist acts out destructively. Carpy (1989) empha-sized that the therapist's partial enactment of the patient's pro-jected contents is what allows patients to observe, consciously or unconsciously, what they cannot tolerate within themselves and therefore have to disavow projectively. By *tolerating* the counter-transference, therapists promote intrapsychic change. Patients see their therapist bearing affective states that the patients have not been able to endure themselves. These observations make the feelings less intolerable and pave the way for the reintrojection of the projected contents *along with* the therapist's capacity to tolerate what previously has been intolerable.

A crucial component of the therapist's holding action is the postponement of interpretation. Projective identification is designed to disavow ownership of certain unacceptable aspects of the self. If the therapist attempts to force the projected contents back into the patient prematurely, the patient will not be able to acknowledge ownership. On the other hand, therapists who can contain what has been projected and tolerate the countertransference provide an opportunity for patients to begin to recognize a part of themselves in the therapist. Carpy (1989) made the following observation: "The analyst's tolerating the countertransference involves his making links in *his* mind, and it is this which allows the patient to do likewise" (p. 293). To become meaningful, interpretations must be delivered *after* patients have recognized parts of themselves in the therapist. Blechner (1992) emphasized that the metabolizing and processing of a projection is done in collaboration with the patient—not unilaterally by the therapist. Premature interpretations of the patient's perception as a projection will only exacerbate defensiveness and paralyze the patient's own attempts to process the projections.

Implicit in this discussion is the notion that patients use the therapist to reclaim aspects of themselves that have been disavowed (Bollas 1989; Scharff 1992). Borderline patients, in particular, attempt to coerce the therapist into becoming someone else. To be therapeutically useful, therapists must meet the patient halfway. They must allow themselves to be transformed sufficiently so that an old relationship is reactivated while maintaining enough of themselves that a new relationship is also being presented. These transference-countertransference enactments re-create an object relationship that may have been largely unconscious for the patient. By examining what is being re-created, the therapist helps the patient translate a largely affective and unconscious experience into conscious and ideational representations that can be analyzed and understood (Bollas 1989). Through appropriate management of countertransference, therapists lead the patient on a journey of discovery. As Bollas (1989) put it: "We need the object to release our self into expression" (p. 48).

The therapist's durability is of the utmost importance in the patient's process of self-discovery. Despite the full destructive force of the patient's transference, the therapist remains indestructible. When patients find that the therapist's ego boundaries are not easily eroded, their own ego boundaries become strengthened as a result. Similarly, they find themselves able to tolerate frustration and contain their own unpleasant feelings rather than having to project them (Epstein 1979).

Therapeutic Disillusionment

In speaking of the mother-infant relationship, Winnicott (1953) observed, "This problem, which undoubtedly concerns the human infant in a hidden way at the beginning, gradually becomes an obvious problem on account of the fact that the mother's main task (next to providing opportunity for illusion) is disillusionment" (p. 95). This paradoxical statement is equally true of psychotherapy—the therapist creates an opportunity for illusion only ultimately to disappoint the patient. Hopes are raised only to be dashed. The creation of the analytic space is an invitation for the patient to re-create old object relationships along with the hope of receiving the gratification that was desired but unobtainable during childhood. The therapist must then frustrate rather than gratify those infantile desires as a way of initiating a mourning process. Only through mourning can the old objects be relinquished.

As we have illustrated in numerous vignettes throughout this volume, the ongoing temptation in the psychotherapy of borderline patients is to try to provide gratification for longings that cannot possibly be satisfied in a professional relationship. Indulging the patient's wishes is a strategy bound to fail and also bound to engender regression by reinforcing infantile expectations, which will only intensify the patient's eventual rage.

When therapists can harness their countertransference wishes to rescue and their feelings of guilt and anger evoked by the patient's demands, they can promote an opportunity for growth and ego-strengthening through the mourning process. Firm boundaries and reasonable limits will eventually reduce the patient's infantile demands. When the therapist refuses to be the idealized, perfect parent, patients will ultimately learn that they must become their own mothers—the wish to fuse and to be fed must be turned inward.

One of the most therapeutic aspects of countertransference management is the therapist's persistent thwarting of the patient's effort to transform the therapist into the all-gratifying parent. In the following vignette the patient attempts to get her therapist into that role by invoking her last therapist.

> Two months into psychotherapy with Dr. B, Ms. Y came to a session and explained in great detail how she had stabbed herself with scissors in her previous therapist's office. Following this harrowing account, the patient asked Dr. B if she could increase her therapy from three to four times per week. She explained that her previous therapist had complied with this request, and it had greatly benefited the therapy.
>
> *Dr. B:* You saw your previous therapist four times a week, and that worked in some ways, but apparently it didn't work in others. In some ways you would like for me to be exactly like her, and in other ways you are terrified that I will be.
> *Ms. Y:* Oh no, I'm not terrified of that. I wish you could be like her. In fact, I just wrote her a long letter telling her about how I'm doing.
>
> Ms. Y then proceeded to read a lengthy communication she had written to her previous therapist in which she talked about her wish to be special. She noted that Dr. B was pretty and friendly but not too helpful. She also asked her previous therapist if she would be available to her in the future after finishing work with Dr. B.
> Dr. B became annoyed with Ms. Y's constant comparison of Dr. B with her previous treater. The thought crossed Dr. B's mind that maybe Ms. Y would shut up about these constant comparisons if she just went ahead and gratified the patient's wish for a fourth appointment per week. However, she chose to contain such feelings and continue to listen. Following the reading of the letter, the

patient discussed at greater length her wish to be special. When the session came to an end and Dr. B had still not acceded to her request for four sessions a week, Ms. Y exploded at her in frustration and slammed the door behind her as she left the office.

When the next session began, Dr. B informed Ms. Y that she would be taking a week's vacation in approximately 1 month.

Ms. Y: Okay, thanks for telling me. I really feel that nobody understands me. I may as well kill myself because I think it's hopeless to ever be understood by another person.

Dr. B felt increasingly angry as Ms. Y continued her wallowing in suicidal wishes. She made numerous efforts to engage Ms. Y in a collaborative discussion about how she could deal with the suicidal thoughts, but the patient simply deflected her efforts and became more sullen. Dr. B eventually noted that nothing she could do or say would be perceived as helpful. Several minutes before the end of the session, Ms. Y brought up her wish to be seen four times a week. When Dr. B again approached the request by inviting further exploration about it, Ms. Y angrily stormed out of the office.

At the next session Ms. Y began by saying that nobody seemed to listen to her when she said what she needed. She indicated that she left Dr. B's office because she was not listening.

Dr. B: I think the question here is whether you can communicate in words rather than actions. When I don't immediately respond to what you want, you use actions to deal with the strong feelings that arise. Instead of leaving my office, I'd like you to tell me what you're feeling.

Ms. Y: I feel so helpless. Nobody listens to me. Nobody cares. I may not come to my next appointment.

The therapist began to feel anxious that the patient's agitation and hopelessness might lead to a suicide attempt. She again felt compelled to respond to the patient's pressures to be the perfect therapist by gratifying the wish for more frequent sessions, but she opted to contain rather than act on her feelings.

Dr. B: I have faith that you will come back even though you're having a hard time now. Thanks for explaining to me where things are. I'll be here on Tuesday.

On Tuesday the patient showed up as expected for her next session.

Ms. Y: I called my previous therapist last week, and she told me to stop fighting with you about meeting more often. She said that such fighting was preventing me from making use of the therapy. I'm getting worse instead of better.

Dr. B: I agree with what your previous therapist said. So much talk about meeting four times a week prevents you from talking about how you're feeling. The purpose of treatment really isn't to make you feel perfect, because that would set you up for disappointment. And I can't be the perfect therapist. You'll always be disappointed in me if that's what you're expecting.

Although the patient appeared to grasp the significance of these statements intellectually, she got more and more agitated. She went on to comment about how her parents had expected her to be perfect as a child and how she had always fallen short of that. Although she was upset at the therapist's limit setting, she stayed for the rest of the session.

The tendency of borderline patients to challenge limits requires the therapist's ongoing vigilance. Even when a contractual understanding has been clearly agreed on during the initial consultations prior to therapy, these patients are likely to test the limits of the contract throughout the course of the psychotherapy. Dr. B's management of her countertransference with Ms. Y, and specifically her ability to resist the temptation to become the perfect, gratifying therapist was clearly in Ms. Y's best interests. By supplying patients what they *need* instead of what they *want,* therapists of borderline patients will ultimately promote greater change.

The Wish to Cure

In discussing the management of countertransference with borderline patients, what the therapist does *not* do is at least as important as what the therapist does. In this regard, one key to therapeutic success is to avoid excessive therapeutic zeal. Paradoxically, the therapist who most wishes to change the patient is the therapist who is least likely to do so. Few borderline patients enlist the therapist's help with the genuine wish to change themselves. Most are consciously or unconsciously invested in changing others so that their own wishes are gratified.

Therapists who approach borderline patients by consistently conveying that change is necessary are likely to be experienced as threatening and unempathic. Patients are likely to feel that the way they *are* is not acceptable to the therapist. The wish to cure the patient is often determined, in part, by a projective identification process in which the therapist has become like the patient's parents, who often have demanded change without taking into account the patient's internal experience. Moreover, the patient may construe any improvement in the therapy as signifying a threat of abandonment (Masterson 1976). From the patient's perspective, the attachment to a reliable and secure person in a quasi-permanent relationship may be of much greater importance than clinical improvement.

In writing about borderline and other difficult patients, Garcia-Badaracco (1992) spoke of the patient as "a specialist in non-change" (p. 210). These patients often feel trapped in a pathological world of internal object relatedness. No matter how miserable they feel, the devil they know may be preferred to the devil they don't know. With any disruption of their ties to problematic internal objects, they face the prospect of abandonment and disconnection and its associated meaninglessness (Gabbard 1989).

To promote therapeutic change, then, the therapist's optimal strategy in psychotherapy with borderline patients is to try to understand and empathize rather than to become a cheerleader who says to the patient, "Come on, you can do it. I know you can." Similarly, therapists who give their borderline patients feedback on how much progress they are making are playing with fire. Many borderline patients hear these attempts at positive reinforcement as indications that the therapy is about to end at any moment. These kinds of communications may then precipitate deteriorating spirals of acting-out behavior to demonstrate to the therapist that the patient is not ready for termination. The ensuing clinical example illustrates this pattern:

> Mr. F was hospitalized with suicidal depression that seemed chronic and intractable. He came into Dr. S's office for psychotherapy one day and said he was furious at his hospital doctor because she said he was getting better. Mr. F maintained emphatically that he was not the slightest bit better.

> *Dr. S:* I guess I'm wondering if you're trying to tell me something about our relationship by complaining about your hospital doctor.
> *Mr. F:* I suppose that's possible. What did you have in mind?
> *Dr. S:* Well, I remember your comment that you felt pretty good the first few days I was gone on my vacation and then felt much worse as I was about to return. I'm wondering if you're worrying about my upcoming vacation again. Can you risk doing well while I'm away?
> *Mr. F:* I get the feeling that if I do better in any way, people think I don't need treatment anymore. You feel you can go on vacation and not have to worry about me.
> *Dr. S:* I know what you mean, but getting better is *not* equal to abandonment. Getting better *is* equivalent to achieving the capacity to give and take. I know that giving has brought risks and difficulties for you.
> *Mr. F:* Where'd you get that idea?

> Dr. S could see that her comment had hurt Mr. F's feelings. She felt badly that she had not been more empathic. Near the end of the session she once again broached the subject of the patient's improvement.

> *Dr. S:* I do think you're getting better, just like your hospital doctor said, but at the same time I can see that you have strong and distressing feelings. Both things can be true. You look more solid now than you did at the beginning of the session.

> Dr. S realized that as soon as the words were out of her mouth, she had once again failed to "tune in" to Mr. F's internal state. He looked dejected and made the following comments right before the end of the hour:

Mr. F: I feel rotten. I don't think I'm going to any of my activities or to team meeting today. I'm just going to stay in bed.

When Mr. F came to his next therapy session, his eyes looked red and swollen, as though he had been crying.

Mr. F: I feel like I'm going psychotic. Everything out there looks horrible. I'm afraid to leave the hospital. You don't believe me. My hospital doctor doesn't believe me. I just can't change. I don't see any reason to live if I always have to live like this.

Mr. F continued to devalue himself and all the treatment he had received from a long series of treaters.

Dr. S: Somehow I feel like I'm being punished, but I don't know why. I think you're trying to communicate something to me, but I can't figure out what it is.

Mr. F: I'm realizing that my condition is serious and chronic. I wish I could just remember some trauma in my past and then undo it. But since I can't remember anything that might have caused all this, I feel hopeless. Being alcoholic doesn't help things. My alcoholism counselor keeps telling me I've got to do Step One.

Mr. F's hopelessness was beginning to engulf Dr. S, who felt a sense of despair about the patient's prognosis. She thought it was important for her to offer some hope to Mr. F.

Dr. S: I agree with your alcoholism counselor, and I also think you need to take Step One here in psychotherapy.

Mr. F: The idea of taking Step One disgusts me. I hate the idea of "once an alcoholic, always an alcoholic." My problems are special and unique. I think I'm really psychotic.

Dr. S: I don't think you're psychotic. I simply think you have feelings that often boil over.

Mr. F: You don't know! You have no idea what's going on inside me!

At the beginning of the next psychotherapy session, Mr. F said he wished to die passively. Maybe if he starved himself, then God would let him into heaven. If he actively killed himself, he speculated, then God would make him go to hell. Dr. S felt that Mr. F's constant focus on suicide and death was oppressive. There seemed to be no way to speak of anything else.

Dr. S: It sounds like you feel the only way to get to heaven is to be self-destructive, but not suicidal.

Mr. F: Yes, of course. I can't go on like this.

In the course of further comments, Mr. F said he felt certain that therapy would not work. Dr. S realized that this determination to defeat the therapy elicited a cheerleader role in her to try to give Mr. F reason for hope and optimism. Rather than continuing to play the role, she reflected back to Mr. F what was happening.

Dr. S: It seems to me that as long you're determined that therapy will not help, it puts me in a position of trying to carry enough hope for both of us and give you reason for optimism.

The case of Mr. F demonstrates how certain borderline patients will actively, although unconsciously, spoil any effort by the therapist or other treaters to suggest that improvement has occurred. The assumption of a thwarting posture vis-à-vis all treaters elicits an encouraging response from the therapist that the patient hears as unempathic. Rather than validating the internal experience of Mr. F, Dr. S reassured him that he was not really psychotic and needed to take "Step One." Many borderline patients coerce hopeful and encouraging responses by asserting complete hopelessness. They then take secret pleasure in defeating and spoiling the therapist's optimistic prognosis (Gabbard 1989). Many of these patients are seeking revenge unconsciously against parents who drove them to do things they did not want to do. Once again, attention to the countertransference pull to become a "cheerleader" may prevent endless repetitions of this cyclic pattern.

Termination

When considering the difficulties that psychotherapists are likely to encounter when facing the termination of a long psychotherapy process, we must keep in mind that many borderline patients live with a sense of dread that they are about to be abandoned by significant others at any moment (Rinsley 1989). Maintaining connectedness with the therapist is often far more important than clinical improvement. These patients are likely to study the therapist's non-verbal communications with extraordinary attention to any clue that might reflect that the therapist is getting fed up with the patient. Indeed, borderline patients can be so exasperating that numerous times in the course of a long treatment the therapist consciously may wish to be rid of the patient. This combination of countertransference, the therapist's exasperation, and the patient's hypervigilance to rejection creates a volatile situation.

Given these dynamics, a useful rule of thumb (although not applicable in all situations) is to let the patient be the first member of the dyad to bring up termination issues. Mismanagement of the countertransference around the time of termination can lead to premature disruption of the therapist-patient bond that will jeopardize the psychological gains of the therapy or to prolonged infantilization that will cause a failure to recognize the patient's increasing need for autonomy. Allowing the patient to set the pace may help guard against either extreme. When allowed to set their own pace, some patients will prefer to draw out the termination phase by gradually diminishing the frequency of sessions over a considerable period so they can "wean" themselves from the therapist.

Whatever termination arrangement is agreed on by patient and therapist, one can predict that things will not proceed smoothly. Many patients abruptly quit therapy. In Waldinger and Gunderson's (1987) study of completed cases with experienced therapists, only about one-third of their sample successfully completed treatment from the perspective of the therapist. Many borderline patients "spoil" the termination process as a way of avoiding the grief associated with the loss of the therapist and the anxiety connected with being on their own. Therapists can find themselves left with an unsatisfying sense that there is unfinished business. By refusing to return for further processing of the abrupt discontinuance, the patient can leave an unmetabolized projection in the therapist that keeps the therapist thinking about the patient (Gabbard 1982). Therapists in such situations find themselves preoccupied with the patient and wondering what went wrong in the process. When this unmetabolized projection gets under the therapist's skin, we can understand it as the patient's unconscious attempt to maintain connectedness with the therapist and thereby deny termination.

Other patients will start "forgetting" appointments. When they do show up for therapy, they will often deny that they are feeling much of anything about the discontinuation of therapy. Many borderline patients with poorly developed object constancy have trouble keeping an image of others in mind when separated. They thus may fear that the therapist will similarly be likely to forget them when they are not in the office together—"out of sight, out of mind." By "forgetting" sessions, these patients actively master a passively experienced trauma through reversal. In other words, they can unconsciously reassure themselves that *they* are the ones doing the forgetting, not the therapist. The fear of being forgotten is thus projected into the therapist, who conveys concern that the patient cannot seem to remember their appointment times. In a similar vein, patients may deny any particular emotional difficulty with the prospect of termination and project all their anxiety into the therapist who grows increasingly distressed at the spotty nature of the patient's attendance.

Those patients who do engage in a serious termination process with the therapist often complain of having lost a certain passion in their lives. If the psychotherapy has gone well, and they have mourned the loss of dreams that can never be fulfilled, they have relinquished infantile claims charged with manic excitement and fantasies of fusion with an omnipotent parent who will make all pain and anxiety disappear. The rewards of reality may seem pallid in comparison with the fantastic expectations with which they entered treatment.

Finally, another subgroup of patients will view the prospect of losing the therapist as so catastrophic that they will escalate acting-out behavior to convince their therapist that termination is ill-advised. Therapists who attempt to treat borderline patients must resign themselves to the fact that certain patients will be "lifers." Wallerstein's (1986) research is encouraging in this regard in that he clearly documented that many patients actually function quite well as long as they can look forward to an occasional contact with the therapist. One final aspect of the management of countertransference is for therapists to accept with equanimity that some patients may become permanent fixtures in their lives.

Summary

The management of countertransference with borderline patients has a therapeutic effect in and of itself. It creates a holding environment in which the patient can internalize a new form of interpersonal relatedness. Optimal containment also provides patients the opportunity to recognize aspects of themselves within the therapist so that when interpretations are ultimately brought to bear, patients can accept them and benefit from them with less defensiveness. Moreover, by attending to the therapeutic frame and the requisite professional boundaries of effective psychotherapy, the therapist facilitates a necessary disillusionment in concert with a mourning process.

Termination is a particularly difficult phase of psychotherapy for borderline patients. The prospect of ending the therapy reawakens the separation and abandonment themes that are central to borderline psychopathology. Allowing the patient to take the lead and set the pace is useful in this regard. Therapists must also be aware that termination is unlikely to proceed smoothly. Some patients may flee the therapy prematurely to avoid the pain of the process; others may turn out to be therapeutic "lifers" who can function adequately only as long as the therapist is available to them.

References

Blechner MJ: Working in the countertransference. Psychoanalytic Dialogues 2:161–179, 1992

Bollas C: Forces of Destiny: Psychoanalysis and Human Idiom. Northvale, NJ, Jason Aronson, 1989

Carpy DV: Tolerating the countertransference: a mutative process. Int J Psychoanal 70:287–294, 1989

Cooper AM: Our changing views of the therapeutic action of psychoanalysis: comparing Strachey and Loewald. Psychoanal Q 57:15–27, 1988

Cooper AM: Psychic change: development in the theory of psychoanalytic techniques. Int J Psychoanal 73:245–250, 1992

Epstein L: Countertransference with borderline patients, in Countertransference: The Therapist's Contribution to the Therapeutic Situation. Edited by Epstein L, Feiner AH. New York, Jason Aronson, 1979, pp 375–405

Gabbard GO: The exit line: heightened transference-countertransference manifestations at the end of the hour. J Am Psychoanal Assoc 30:579–598, 1982

Gabbard GO: Patients who hate. Psychiatry 52:96–106, 1989

Gabbard GO: Psychodynamic Psychiatry in Clinical Practice: The DSM-IV Edition. Washington, DC, American Psychiatric Press, 1994

Gabbard GO, Horwitz L, Frieswyk S, et al: The effect of therapist interventions on the therapeutic alliance with borderline patients. J Am Psychoanal Assoc 36:697–727, 1988

Garcia-Badaracco JE: Psychic change and its clinical evaluation. Int J Psychoanal 73:209–220, 1992

Hamilton NG: Self and Others: Object Relations Theory in Practice. Northvale, NJ, Jason Aronson, 1988

Horwitz L: Clinical Prediction in Psychotherapy. New York, Jason Aronson, 1974

Loewald HW: On the therapeutic action of psychoanalysis (1960), in Papers on Psychoanalysis. New Haven, CT, Yale University Press, 1980, pp 221–256

Luborsky L: Principles in Psychoanalytic Therapy: A Manual for Supportive-Expressive Treatment. New York, Basic Books, 1984

Masterson JF: Psychotherapy of the Borderline Adult: A Developmental Approach. New York, Brunner/Mazel, 1976

Meissner WW: Treatment of Patients in the Borderline Spectrum. Northvale, NJ, Jason Aronson, 1988

Meissner WW: What Is Effective in Psychoanalytic Therapy: The Move From Interpretation to Relation. Northvale, NJ, Jason Aronson, 1991

Ogden TH: On projective identification. Int J Psychoanal 60:357–373, 1979

Ogden TH: The Matrix of the Mind: Object Relations and the Psychoanalytic Dialogue. Northvale, NJ, Jason Aronson, 1986

Ogden TH: The Primitive Edge of Experience. Northvale, NJ, Jason Aronson, 1989

Pulver SE: Psychic change: insight or relationship? Int J Psychoanal 73:199–208, 1992

Rinsley DB: Developmental Pathogenesis and Psychoanalytic Treatment of Borderline and Narcissistic Personalities. Northvale, NJ, Jason Aronson, 1989

Rockland LH: Supportive Therapy for Borderline Patients: A Psychodynamic Approach. New York, Guilford, 1992

Scharff DE: Refinding the Object and Reclaiming the Self. Northvale, NJ, Jason Aronson, 1992

Strachey J: The nature of the therapeutic action of psycho-analysis. Int J Psychoanal 15:127–159, 1934

Waldinger RJ, Gunderson JG: Effective Psychotherapy With Borderline Patients: Case Studies. New York, MacMillan, 1987

Wallerstein RS: Forty-Two Lives in Treatment: A Study of Psychoanalysis and Psychotherapy. New York, Guilford, 1986

Winnicott DW: Transitional objects and transitional phenomena: a study of the first not-me possession. Int J Psychoanal 34:89–97, 1953

Index